5 INGREDIENT DIABETIC DIET COOKBOOK FOR BEGINNERS

$10/MEAL OR LESS

60-DAY MEAL PLAN

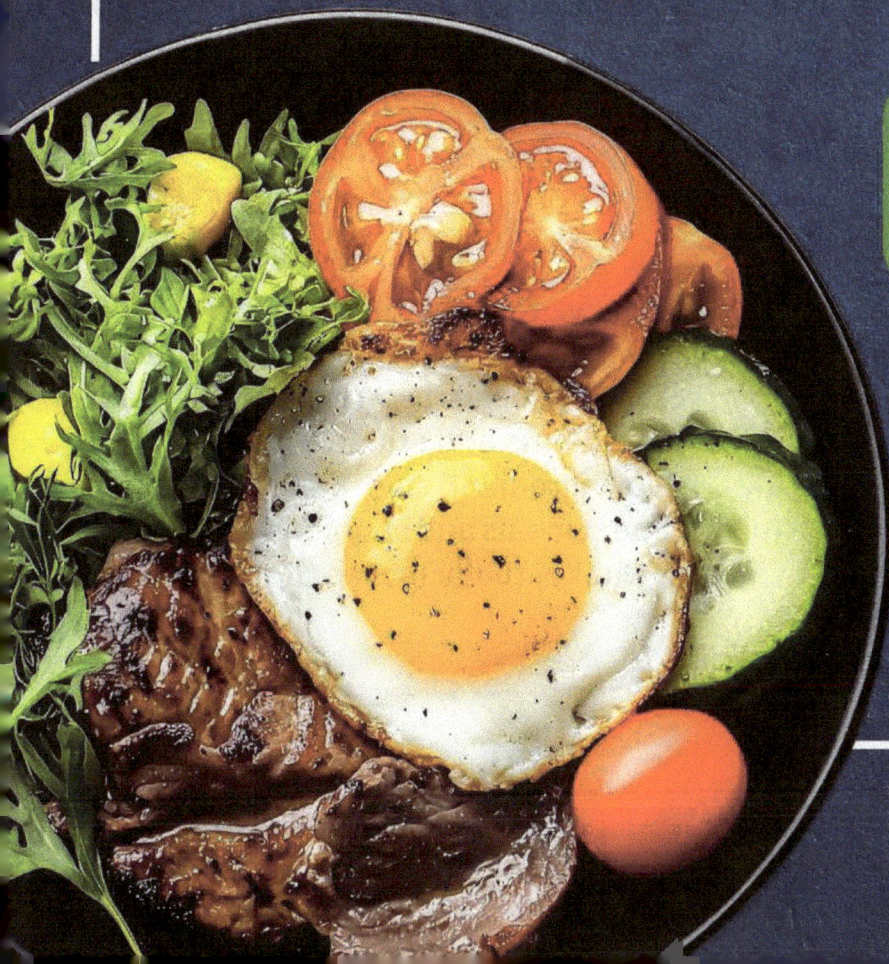

DIETITIAN APPROVED ✓

FULL COLOR

ELIZABETH M. BERKEY
MARIANNE GREENE

Praise

Most people with type 2 diabetes do not struggle because they lack motivation. They struggle because the plan is too complicated. This cookbook removes that barrier. Five ingredients per recipe, quick cook times, and a realistic budget focus make it truly doable. I also appreciate the practical structure. Clear portions, consistent meal timing, and meals built around fiber and protein can support steadier post meal numbers."

— Elena P., Registered Dietitian Nutritionist (RDN)

"As a primary care physician, I am always looking for resources that help patients turn guidance into real meals. This book does that. The 60 day plan reduces decision fatigue, the recipes are simple enough for true beginners, and the under $10 approach meets people where they are financially. It is the kind of guide that helps patients build habits, not just cook a few recipes."

— Maya S., MD

"I have tried diabetic cookbooks that assume you have a gourmet kitchen, specialty ingredients, and endless time. This one is refreshingly real. I can shop once, cook fast, and still enjoy food that feels normal. The recipes are simple, but the results are flavorful, and I do not feel like I am dieting."

— Carlos M., Type 2 Diabetes Patient

"The best part is how beginner friendly it is. The grocery lists are short, the steps are clear, and everything actually fits into my day. I prep in under 30 minutes, pack leftovers for lunch, and I am not constantly guessing what to eat next. The meal plan is a lifesaver."

— Tiffany R., Busy Parent and Meal Prep Newbie

"This cookbook hits the sweet spot for blood sugar supportive eating. Simple carbs are kept in check, meals emphasize non starchy vegetables, lean proteins, and satisfying fats, and portions make sense. It is a strong starting point for anyone newly diagnosed who needs a straightforward plan they can stick to."

— Jordan K., Certified Diabetes Care and Education Specialist (CDCES)

"Finally, recipes that do not rely on expensive diet products. I appreciate that the meals use regular, affordable ingredients and still feel complete. The five ingredient rule makes it easy to repeat meals and stay consistent, which is what actually moves the needle over time."

— Priya D., Budget Conscious Home Cook

Disclaimer and Legal Notice

Table of Contents

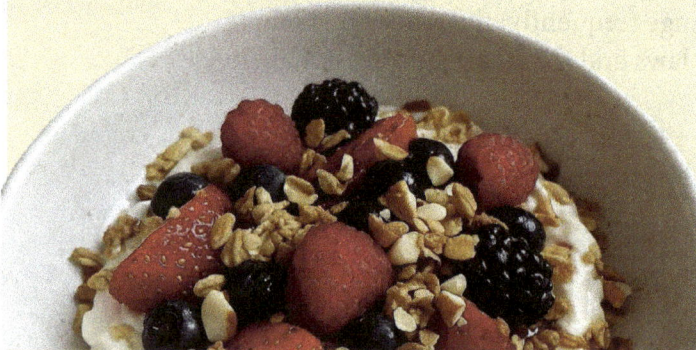

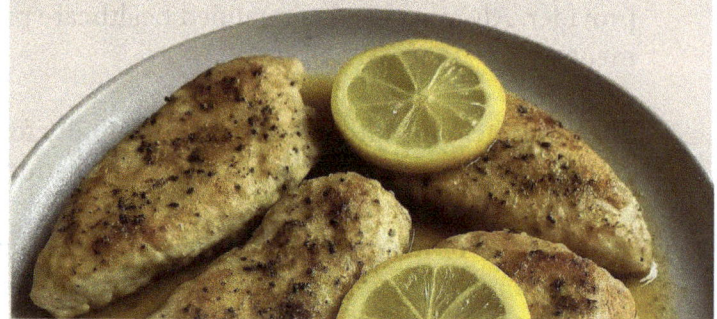

Table of Contents

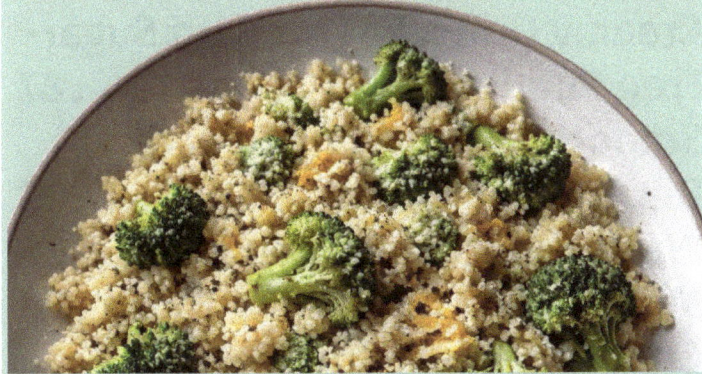

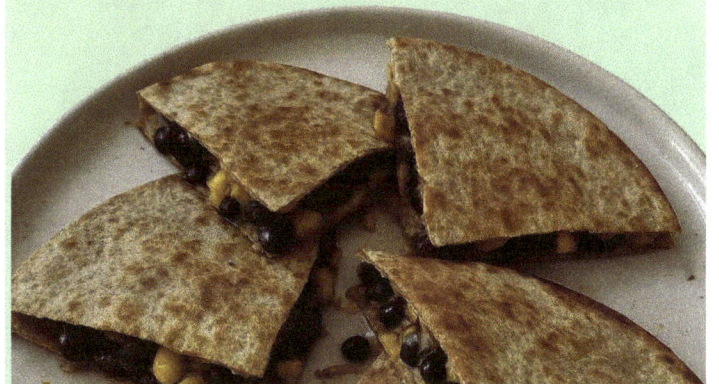

Table of Contents

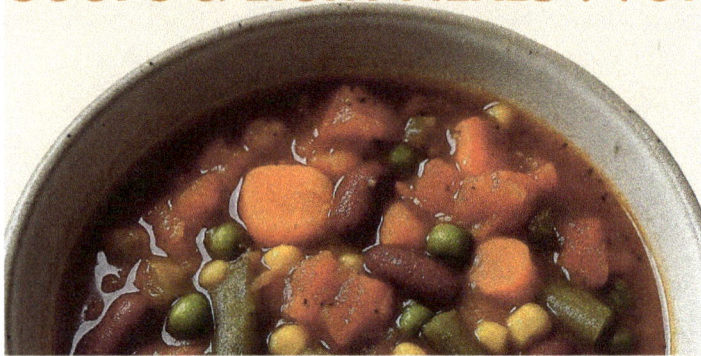

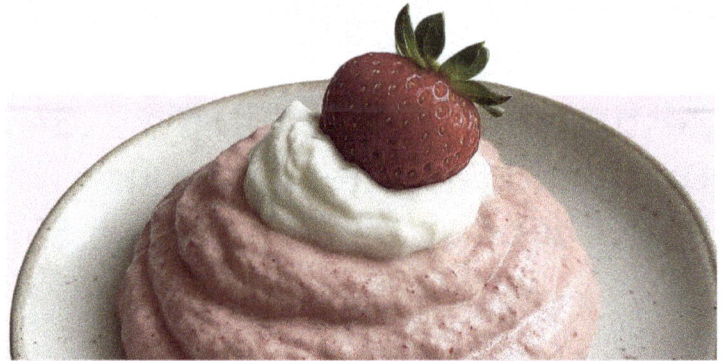

Don't forget your bonuses

These tools come in handy:

◊ Avoid Sugar Spikes – Carb Swap Cheat Sheet (PDF)

◊ DIY Meal Planner – make your own plan & adjust recipes (Printable PDF)

◊ 11 Tips for Staying Active Safely With Diabetes (PDF)

◊ Information about becoming an advance reader for our next book

The Bonus section is listed at the end of the Table of Contents

All bonuses are optional and waiting for you when you're ready.

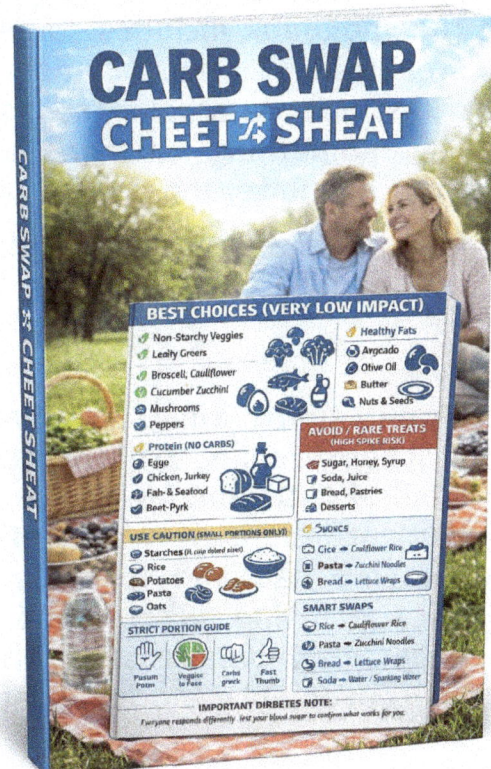

Cookbook Introduction:

Quick and affordable meals for Type 2 diabetes management

Living with type 2 diabetes does not mean giving up the foods you love; it means learning how to support your body with meals that keep you full, energized, and satisfied.

This cookbook was designed for busy adults who want simple, affordable 5-ingredient meals, ready in 30 minutes or less, and under $10 per recipe.

Whether you were recently diagnosed or returning to healthy habits, this guide will help make eating with diabetes easier, not harder.

Inside, you'll find 60 delicious and realistic diabetes-friendly recipes that are comforting, affordable, and fast to prepare.

The cookbook includes soups, salads, breakfasts, lunches, dinners, snacks, fruits, and desserts — so you always have something satisfying to choose from, no matter the time of day.

A 60-day easy-to-use meal plan is also included.

Why I Became a Dietitian

My nutrition journey started while I was in school, training to become a Certified Medical Assistant. I was working in our student laboratory when I discovered that my dad had diabetes. He was already living with heart disease, juggling a high-stress job, and relying on convenience foods to get through

long days. That lab result didn't just belong to a patient; it belonged to my dad. And in that moment, everything changed.

I realized I didn't want to work as an assistant to a physician simply. I wanted to be the person physicians referred to for expertise in nutrition, someone who takes a direct and meaningful role in patient care and helps people long before things become overwhelming.

Becoming a dietitian allowed me to combine clinical knowledge with compassion, and to give people, as well as my dad, the tools they needed to take control of their health. It became my purpose to provide guidance that is realistic, supportive, and practical, not stressful or confusing.

Every time I work with a patient, I'm reminded of why I chose this path.

My career is more than a profession; it is a mission rooted in love, experience, and the belief that everyone deserves knowledge, support, and hope.

Why I Co-Authored this Cookbook

I've been a Registered Dietitian Nutritionist for more than 25 years, specializing in diabetes care, and throughout my career, I've met countless patients who were trying their hardest but still struggling with diet and meal planning. They worked long hours, skipped meals, picked up whatever was convenient, and felt like they were constantly "starting over." It wasn't that they didn't want to be healthy; they simply didn't have guidance that fit real life.

So many people were told what not to eat, but no one showed them what a realistic diabetes-friendly meal actually looks like, with steady, predictable carbohydrates, fiber, and lean protein that help blood sugar rise gently and settle back down again. On top of that, the world is flooded with fad diets, conflicting nutrition advice, and misinformation. Patients are left confused, overwhelmed, and unsure who to trust. Many believe eating for diabetes means perfection, sacrifice, and giving up the foods they love, instead of feeling satisfied, supported, and in control.

Seeing so many individuals with diabetes struggle made something very clear to me: people don't fail because they lack willpower. They struggle because they aren't given simple, practical tools that make everyday eating easier. I wanted to create a resource that replaces stress and confusion with confidence and relief, one that feels doable on the busiest days, not just the perfect ones.

That's why this cookbook exists.

Every recipe in this book was designed for real-life, comforting, familiar meals with balanced carbohydrates, high fiber, and lean protein that support blood sugar without feeling like a diet. No judgment. No fear. No complicated rules.

Just approachable meals that help you feel good today while supporting better A1C, energy, and health over time. Because diabetes management shouldn't feel overwhelming, it should feel possible.

Understanding Type 2 Diabetes

Type 2 diabetes occurs when the body does not use insulin effectively or does not make enough insulin.

When insulin cannot do its job, glucose builds up in the bloodstream instead of entering the cells for energy[1].

Navigating diabetes is not about avoiding carbohydrates or being perfect. It is about:

◊ **Eating balanced meals on a predictable schedule**

◊ **Supporting your body with foods that promote steady energy**

◊ **Developing realistic routines you can follow consistently**

Balanced nutrition, regular movement, stress management, adequate sleep, and medication (when needed) all work together to support health.

You don't have to do everything at once; small changes add up.

Why Blood Sugar Control Matters

Keeping blood sugar steady can dramatically improve how you feel day-to-day and protect long-term health[1].

A steady blood sugar can:

◊ **Improve energy and stamina**

◊ **Support mood and mental clarity**

◊ **Reduce cravings and hunger swings**

◊ **Support healthy metabolism and**

weight

◊ Protect the heart, kidneys, nerves, and eyes

◊ Improve sleep and overall quality of life

Managing blood sugar is not about restriction; it's about empowerment.

What is A1C and FBG

Before we talk about how Type 2 diabetes is diagnosed, it helps to understand two important numbers you will hear often: A1C and fasting glucose.

A1C

Your A1C shows your average blood sugar over the past 2 to 3 months.

An easy way to think about it is like your credit score. It does not show what you spent today. It shows your overall habits over time. Even if you have a few good or bad days, the A1C looks at the bigger picture.

Fasting Glucose

Your fasting glucose is your blood sugar first thing in the morning, before you eat.

This is like checking the fuel level in your car before you start driving for the day. It tells you where things stand before food or activity changes anything.

Together, these numbers help you and your healthcare team understand how your body is handling sugar and what steps can support better health.

Diagnosing Type 2 Diabetes

Type 2 diabetes is diagnosed through blood tests that measure how the body processes glucose. A diagnosis is typically made when fasting blood glucose is 126 mg/dL or higher, A1C is 6.5% or higher, or a 2-hour glucose tolerance test result is 200 mg/dL or higher.

In some cases, a random blood glucose test result of 200 mg/dL or higher, accompanied by symptoms, can also indicate diabetes.

Results below these levels, such as an A1C between 5.7% and 6.4% indicate a prediabetes range, meaning blood sugar is higher than normal but not yet in the diabetes range.

Regardless of where someone starts, nutrition plays a crucial role in preventing progression, supporting stable blood sugar levels, and promoting long-term health.

Blood Sugar Control in Diabetes

Good blood-sugar control means keeping glucose levels within a healthy range throughout the day, not too high and not too low.

◊ For most adults with Type 2 diabetes, this includes a fasting blood sugar around 80–130 mg/dL first thing in the morning.

◊ Staying under 180 mg/dL about 1–2 hours after meals (your provider may set individual targets)2.

Consistent, balanced meals spaced every 3–5 hours, including lean protein, high-fiber carbs, vegetables, and healthy fats; and limiting added sugars helps prevent sharp spikes and crashes.

The goal isn't perfection, it's steady, predictable glucose levels that keep you energized, protect your heart, eyes, nerves, and kidneys, and help you feel your best every day.

How Blood Sugar Affects the Way You Feel

Blood sugar isn't just a lab number; it influences how you feel, how you think, how much energy you have, and whether you feel like yourself. So many people assume they're tired, unfocused, moody, or "just having an off day," when in reality their blood sugar is simply out of range. This isn't failure. It's the body asking for support.

When Blood Sugar Is High

High blood sugar can make you feel:

- Thirsty
- Weak
- Headachy
- Extremely hungry
- Tired and worn down
- Foggy or unfocused
- Blurry-eyed

One of my clients, John, experienced this in a very real way. His vision became so blurry that he rushed to get an eye exam and bought new glasses. A few weeks later, once his blood sugar came down, his vision returned to normal, and those new glasses sat unused. What looked like his eyesight getting worse was actually his blood sugar running too high.

What Can Help:

- **Hydration** — when blood sugar is high, the body becomes dehydrated. Drinking 8 oz of water every hour can support the body's natural balancing process.

- **Movement** — even a 10–20 minute walk after a larger meal helps muscles use glucose for energy, reducing the post-meal spike.

- **Balanced fueling** — watching portion sizes and eating consistently throughout the day (instead of skipping meals, then overeating later) helps keep blood sugar from swinging too high.

When Blood Sugar Is Low

- Low blood sugar develops when the body runs out of available glucose, and it can come on fast. Symptoms can include:

- Shakiness
- Sweating
- Sudden hunger
- A racing heartbeat
- Irritability or anxiety
- Trouble thinking clearly
- Dizziness

Low blood sugar is often triggered by skipping meals, eating too few carbohydrates, taking medication without food, exercising more than usual, or drinking alcohol without eating.

One of my clients, Yvonne, thought she was being "disciplined" by drinking coffee all day and only eating dinner.

Instead, her blood sugar kept crashing, leaving her dizzy and frightened. When she learned that carbohydrates paired with protein throughout the day protect her blood sugar, her brain, and her energy, everything changed. She began to feel stable again, mentally, physically, and emotionally.

How to treat low blood sugar: 15/15 rule

1. Take 15 grams of fast-acting carbohydrates (juice, glucose tablets, soda, honey).

2. Wait 15 minutes and recheck blood sugar.

3. Once blood sugar rises to 70 mg/dL on a meter or 80 mg/dL on a CGM, eat a snack with carbohydrates + protein (yogurt and fruit, peanut butter toast, cheese and crackers) to keep levels steady.

The Foundation of Feeling Better

You don't need a perfect diet to feel better; you need consistency.

Most people feel steadier, clearer, and more energized with:

- Three balanced meals per day
- One planned snack (if needed)
- Predictable carbohydrates + lean protein + fiber
- Hydration
- Gentle movement after larger meals

These aren't rules, they're support.

They tell your body: "You're safe. You're being taken care of."

You Deserve to Feel Good

When blood sugar is steadier, people often notice:

- Better mood
- Sharper thinking
- More energy
- Fewer cravings
- Better sleep
- Less anxiety around food
- More confidence and control

A1C Goals: How This Cookbook Can Get You There

Managing diabetes isn't about perfection; it's about progress. One of the most important markers of diabetes control is the A1C, a blood test that reflects your average blood sugar over the past 2–3 months.

According to the American Diabetes Association (ADA), the general A1C goal for most non-pregnant adults is below 7%, unless a different individualized target has been set by a healthcare provider.

Keeping A1C within your personalized goal range reduces the risk of nerve damage, kidney disease, eye complications, and heart disease while supporting long-term energy, mobility, and overall quality of life.

Reaching A1C goals isn't about restriction or giving up favorite foods. It's about learning how to balance meals so your body gets the nutrients it needs without sharp blood sugar spikes. When meals contain balanced carbohydrates, lean protein, fiber-rich vegetables, and heart-healthy fats, blood glucose rises more gently and returns to target more quickly, which, over time, leads to improved A1C results.

One of my patients, Steve, will always stay with me. His A1C had been out of control for years, and both he and his nurse practitioner were frustrated and discouraged. He wasn't lazy, careless, or ignoring advice; he just didn't have the right tools. When he was referred to me for outpatient nutrition counseling, we sat together and broke down what a carbohydrate-balanced pattern of eating actually looks like in real life. I'll never forget the moment his eyes widened, he smiled, and said, "I finally get it." Something that once felt confusing and overwhelming suddenly made sense to him, and you could see the relief in his face.

A few months later, he went back to his NP for repeat labs, and his A1C had dropped to the best level of his entire adult life. His NP even reached out to personally thank me for helping her patient. That was a very good day, not because of the numbers on a chart, but because someone who once felt defeated now felt confident, capable, and in control of his health.

This cookbook is designed to make blood sugar balance simple and realistic. Every recipe supports better A1C control by including:

- ~40–60 grams of carbohydrate per meal, a range that supports steady blood sugars for most adults
- Lean protein to promote fullness and prevent overeating
- High-fiber vegetables and whole grains slow digestion and improve insulin response.
- Lower sodium and lower fat ingredients to support both heart and blood sugar health
- Convenience and affordability, so healthy eating works in real life, not just on perfect days

Whether your goal is to lower your A1C, maintain your progress, or get back on track, the structure of these meals is intentionally designed to help you get there.

You don't have to count every gram or memorize food lists; simply follow the recipes, enjoy the flavors, and let the balance in each dish support your blood sugar and A1C behind the scenes.

Your A1C tells the story of your habits over time. This cookbook is here to help that story become one of confidence, control, and meals you genuinely enjoy.

Importance of Exercise

Exercise is essential for managing diabetes. Muscles use glucose for energy, which can help lower blood sugar and improve blood sugar control. Cells also become more sensitive to insulin.

Exercise can help with weight management and reduce the risk of heart disease[3].

Consult your doctor before beginning any exercise program. Monitor blood sugar before and after exercise to see how it affects you.

Aim for 150 minutes per week of moderate-intensity exercise such as walking (or 30 minutes a day, five days a week).

- Break sessions into 10-minute intervals if needed.

- Exercise can also enhance sleep, improve mood, and boost overall sense of well-being.

- Even little changes can make a big difference.

Heart Healthy Eating

People with diabetes have a higher risk of heart disease, so supporting both blood sugar and heart health is essential[3].

The recipes in this cookbook emphasize:

- Lean proteins (chicken, turkey, fish, eggs, low-fat dairy, lean cuts of pork and beef)

- High-fiber fruits, vegetables, and whole grains

- Healthy fats (plant-based oils, canola, olive, peanut, nuts, avocado, tuna)

- Herbs and spices instead of excess salt

Heart-supportive habits don't have to be dramatic:

- One plant-based meal per week or more can help lower cholesterol

- Adding Omega-3 fatty acids 2–3 times per week can help lower triglycerides[3]

This cookbook is not just about managing the blood sugar; it is also about protecting the heart.

Whether your goal is to lower your A1C, maintain your progress, or get back on track, the structure of these meals is intentionally designed to help you get there.

You don't have to count every gram or memorize food lists; simply follow the recipes, enjoy the flavors, and let the balance in each dish support your blood sugar and A1C behind the scenes.

Your A1C tells the story of your habits over time. This cookbook is here to help that story become one of confidence, control, and meals you genuinely enjoy.

Importance of Exercise

Exercise is essential for managing diabetes. Muscles use glucose for energy, which can help lower blood sugar and improve blood sugar control. Cells also become more sensitive to insulin.

Exercise can help with weight management and reduce the risk of heart disease[3].

Consult your doctor before beginning any exercise program. Monitor blood sugar before and after exercise to see how it affects you.

Aim for 150 minutes per week of moderate-intensity exercise such as walking (or 30 minutes a day, five days a week).

- Break sessions into 10-minute intervals if needed.

- Exercise can also enhance sleep, improve mood, and boost overall sense of well-being.

- Even little changes can make a big difference.

When Alcohol Was the Missing Puzzle Piece

One of my former patients, Michael, taught me a lesson I will never forget, and it's one that many people living with diabetes can relate to. He enjoyed having drinks with friends and didn't think alcohol had anything to do with his blood sugar.

In fact, he assumed it raised his glucose the same way desserts might. What hedidn't realize was that heavy drinking, especially without food, can cause blood sugar to drop hours later, even during sleep.

Michael often drank more than the recommended limit for men, and most of the time he did so on an empty stomach after long workdays. His daytime numbers looked fine, but almost every night he woke up sweating, shaky, and confused.

He kept blaming dinner, exercise, stress, anything he could think of. It never crossed his mind that alcohol could be behind the low blood sugar episodes.

When we reviewed his glucose logs together, a pattern appeared: normal blood sugars in the evening followed by sudden overnight crashes on the nights he drank. He was shocked. No one had ever told him that the liver prioritizes clearing alcohol over releasing stored glucose, meaning alcohol can block the liver from preventing low blood sugar, especially if there is no food on board.

The turning point came when Michael made one simple change: he started eating with his drinks, choosing snacks with carbs + protein, like whole-grain crackers with cheese, yogurt, nuts with fruit, or a small sandwich. He also cut back on how much he drank. The nighttime lows disappeared almost immediately. He wasn't "doing everything wrong"; he simply didn't have the information.

Michael's experience is a reminder that diabetes management isn't about blame; it's about learning what your body needs to stay safe. Sometimes the solution isn't restriction; it's understanding.

Alcohol Guidelines for Diabetes

People with diabetes can include alcohol safely, but it requires planning because alcohol can lower blood sugar, especially when combined with certain diabetes medications.

General safety tips

- Always eat a meal or snack that contains carbohydrates when drinking
- Never drink on an empty stomach, as it raises the risk of low blood sugar
- Monitor blood sugar before bed after drinking
- Wear a medical ID when drinking socially
- Limit intake to moderation:
  - Women: 1 drink per day
  - Men: 2 drinks per day

ALCOHOL CONSUMPTION GUIDELINES

DAILY LIMITS:

MEN:
2 DRINKS PER DAY

WHAT COUNTS AS ONE DRINK?

DRINK	SERVING SIZE
Wine	5 oz
Beer	12 oz
Light beer	12 oz
Liquor (vodka, gin, whiskey, rum, tequila, etc)	1.5 oz

DAILY LIMITS:

WOMEN:
1 DRINKS PER DAY

WHAT COUNTS AS ONE DRINK?

DRINK	SERVING SIZE
Wine	5 oz
Beer	12 oz
Light beer	12 oz
Liquor (vodka, gin, whiskey, rum, tequila, etc)	1.5 oz

Tips By Alcohol Type

Alcohol Type	Diabetes considerations
Wine	Usually does not raise blood sugar sharply, best with food
Beer	Contains carbohydrates, which can raise blood sugar
Light Beer	Low Carb Option
Liquor (plain)	Does not contain carbs, but can cause LOW blood sugar
Mixed drinks/ cocktails	Often high in sugar, use zero-sugar mixers

Better Mixer Choices

- Diet soda
- Club soda
- Sparkling water
- Sugar-free lemonade
- Light cranberry juice (½ cup + water)
- Fresh lemon or lime + soda water

Avoid or Limit

- Regular soda cocktails
- Frozen margaritas, piña coladas
- Sweet wines/dessert wines
- Sugar-laden mixers (energy drinks, regular tonic water)

Safety Note

Low blood sugar from alcohol can occur up to 24 hours later. If you use insulin or sulfonylurea medications, be especially cautious and eat a carbohydrate-containing snack before bed if drinking.

Balanced Meals Work Best

Carbohydrates are not the enemy. Your brain and body require carbohydrates for energy and to function properly. What matters most is the balance of nutrients at each meal and the portion size eaten.

Most Adults Do Well With[1]:

- ~40–60 g of carbohydrates per meal
- Lean protein at each meal
- Fiber from vegetables, whole fruits, legumes, or whole grains
- Healthy fats in moderation over saturated fats

This Combination:

- Slows digestion
- Promotes fullness and satisfaction

- Minimizes blood sugar spikes and crashes

Skipping Meals Often Backfires:

- Blood sugar can spike later in the dayHunger intensifies
- Cravings increase

Most People Feel Their Best With:

- 3 balanced meals daily
- 1 snack if needed (a carbohydrate paired with protein or healthy fat)

This balanced eating pattern aligns with evidence-based nutrition guidelines for diabetes management[1].

Build a ~40-60 gram Carbohydrate Meal:

A balanced plate for diabetes includes carbohydrates + protein + vegetables, + healthy fats.

 Most adults feel their best with ~40–60 grams of carbohydrates per meal, which supports steady energy, fullness, and stable blood sugar.

Use the tables below to mix and match foods to build a blood-sugar-friendly meal, without measuring or calorie counting. A woman's fist or a baseball is about 1 cup.

Step 1 — Choose 1-2 Carbohydrate Portions (30-60 g carb)

Food	Portion	Food	Portion
Brown rice	1 cup / 45 g carbs	Whole-wheat pasta	1 cup cooked / 45 g carbs
Whole-wheat bread	2 slices / 30 g carbs	Oatmeal	1 cup cooked / 30 g carbs
Quinoa	1 cup cooked / 39 g carbs	Whole-wheat tortilla	8-inch / 25 g carbs
English muffin	1 whole / 27 g carbs	Sweet potato	1 medium / 27 g carbs
Corn	1 cup / 30 g carbs	Fruit	1 medium or 1 cup / 15 g carbs

STEP 2 — Choose 1 Lean Protein Portion (~8 grams carbs or less)

Food	Portion Size
Chicken breast	3–4 oz
Turkey	3–4 oz
Tuna (canned or fresh)	3–4 oz
Fish (cod, tilapia, salmon, etc.)	3–4 oz
Eggs	2 eggs
Cottage cheese (higher in sodium)	1 cup
Greek yogurt (plain)	¾ cup
Lean pork or beef	3–4 oz
Tofu	¾ cup

Fuel Your Body Right

Protein helps slow digestion, prevent blood sugar spikes, improve satiety, and support muscle health.

STEP 3 - CHOOSE 1-2 SERVINGS OF NON-STARCHY VEGETABLES

(~5 GRAMS CARB FOR 1/2 CUP COOKED OR 1 CUP RAW)

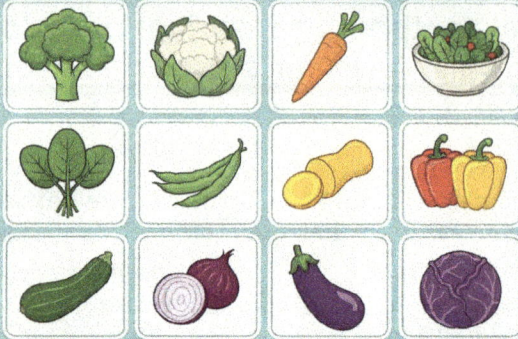

FUEL YOUR BODY RIGHT

DIABETIC FRIENDLY CHOICE

Meal Example	Carbs consideration
1 cup brown rice + 3 oz chicken + 1 cup cooked broccoli	≈ 55 g
1 cup whole-wheat pasta + 3 turkey meat-balls + 1 cup raw spinach	≈ 50 g
2 slices of whole-wheat bread + 2 eggs + 2 cup salad greens	≈ 40 g ≈ 50 g
1 cup quinoa + 3-4 oz salmon + 1 cup cooked green beans	≈ 49 g
1 medium sweet potato + 3-4 oz tuna + 1 cup cooked asparagus	≈ 37 g
1 cup oatmeal + Nonfat, Unsweetened Greek yogurt + ¾ cup blueberries	≈ 52 g
1-8" tortilla + shredded chicken + 1 cup cooked peppers/onions + ½ cup canned peaches	≈ 50 g

Vegetables add fiber, which supports fullness and blood sugar control.

STEP 4 — Include Healthy Fat
(optional but helpful)

Food	Portion
Olive oil or canola oil	1 Tbsp
Avocado	¼–½
Nuts	1 oz
Peanut butter	1–2 Tbsp
Seeds (flax, chia, pumpkin)	1–2 Tbsp
Olives	8–10

Fuel Your Body Right

DIABETIC FRIENDLY CHOICE

Healthy fats help increase meal satisfaction and support heart health; no need to avoid them, just use them in moderation.

EXAMPLE MEAL COMBINATIONS (40–60 g carbs)

Key Takeaways

If your meal includes:

- 1-2 carbohydrate portions (~30-60 g)
- 1 protein
- 1-2 servings of non-starchy vegetables
- Optional healthy fat

This is a very healthy way of eating for long-term health and blood sugar control, and it is sustainable for a lifetime.

How My Dad Taught Me the Power of Small Changes

My work as a Registered Dietitian is inspired in many ways by my dad, who lived with type 2 diabetes and had a lifelong love of sweets. Desserts were his comfort, and at first, he believed diabetes meant he had to give them up forever.

But what changed everything wasn't restriction — it was discovering how to modify his favorite treats so they were diabetes-friendly. By lowering added sugar, increasing fiber, and pairing sweets with protein, he realized he could still enjoy the flavors he loved without causing a sharp rise in blood sugar.

Watching how these small adjustments created big changes — not just in his glucose numbers, but in his confidence, energy, and peace of mind — taught me something important: diabetes care should never take joy away from food. It should give people more ways to live fully, with support, flexibility, and meals that feel familiar, satisfying, and realistic.

My dad always loved making his homemade chocolate fudge. It was his comfort, his reward, and one of his greatest joys, especially after a long week. So when I suggested trying a diabetes-friendly snack instead, he gave me that playful look, the one that said, "Good luck convincing me."

But one summer evening in the kitchen together, instead of making his usual homemade chocolate fudge, I showed him how to make a diabetes-friendly chocolate brownie, something sweet that felt familiar but gentler on his blood sugar. He took a bite, leaned against the counter, and slowly a smile spread across his face. Then he laughed and said,

"It's not the chocolate fudge... but it's pretty good."

It was a sweet moment, but what stayed with me wasn't the joke; it was everything that happened afterward. He didn't feel tired, weak, or guilty. He didn't worry about sugar spikes or whether he had "messed up." He just enjoyed the snack, the warmth of the kitchen, and the moment. He felt good. And I got to witness him simply feel good.

That moment reshaped the way I view diabetes care. It proved that success isn't about perfection, it's about realistic solutions that protect joy. People need foods that make them feel safe and supported, not scared or restricted. They need options that let them still feel like themselves.

That memory stays with me every time I help someone with diabetes. Everyone deserves that same feeling, enjoyment, comfort, and the confidence that they can eat in a way that supports their health without giving up the foods that make life feel full.

Smart Snack Examples For Better Blood Sugar

Snacks work best when they pair carbohydrates + protein or healthy fats to avoid spikes and crashes.

Snack Time Guidance

Snacks are optional, but may help when:

- Blood sugar trends low between meals
- Meals are spaced 5+ hours apart
- You're physically active
- You take insulin or certain diabetes medications

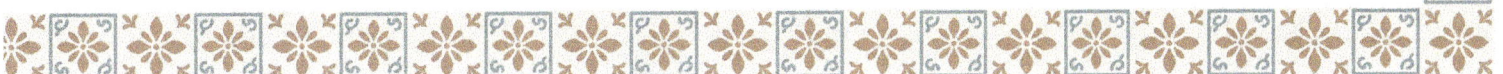

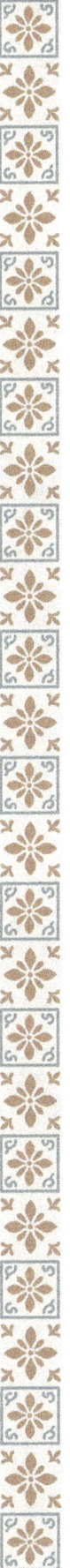

10–15-gram carb snack ideas

Snack	Why it Works
Apple slices + peanut butter	Fiber + protein for steady energy
Cottage cheese + blueberries	High protein + moderate carbs
Greek yogurt (plain) + cinnamon	Protein helps stabilize blood sugar≈ 50 g
Hummus + bell pepper strips	Fiber + plant-based protein
1 hard-boiled egg + 1 small orange	Balanced protein + carb
Whole-grain crackers + cheese	Slow-digesting carbs + fat
Strawberries + almonds	Fiber + healthy fats
Tuna salad on cucumber slices	Protein + zero refined carbs

25–30-gram carb snack ideas (good for active days)

Snack	Why it Works
1 slice whole-grain toast + avocado	Carbs + fiber + healthy fats
Oatmeal packet (plain) + walnuts	Carbs + fat for slow digestion
Banana + 1 Tbsp peanut butter	Balanced carbs + fat
Trail mix without candy	Slow-digesting, portable
Smoothie: milk + spinach + berries	Balanced and nutrient-dense

Quick Snack Formulas for Healthy Snacks

Carbohydrate (10–30 g) + Protein or Healthy Fat = Better blood sugar + Less hunger

Examples:

- Crackers + cheese
- Fruit + nuts
- Yogurt + berries
- Toast + nut butter

Glycemic Index

The glycemic index (GI) is a tool that measures how quickly a carbohydrate raises blood sugar levels, on a scale of 0 to 100.

Foods with a low GI (55 or less) release glucose slowly, while high-GI foods (70 or more) cause rapid fluctuations[2].

Foods low in fiber generally have a higher glycemic index. Pairing high-GI foods with protein and fiber can help slow the digestion of the carbohydrate.

Food Group	Low GI (≤55)	Medium GI (56–69)	High GI (≥70)
Grains & Starcheses	Steel-cut oats (42)	Brown rice (68)	–
	Whole-wheat pasta (41)	Couscous (65)	–
	Quinoa (53)	Whole-wheat pita (57)	–
	Sweet potato, boiled (44)	Instant oatmeal packet (65)	–
Fruits	Apple (36) Orange (43)	Pineapple (59) Banana (62)	Watermelon (76)
	Berries (40)	Raisins (64)	–
	Grapes (53)	Mango (56)	–
Vegetables	Non-starchy vegetables — broccoli, spinach, zucchini, cauliflower (~15)	Sweet corn (60)	French fries (75) Instant mashed potatoes (87)
Dairy & Alternatives	Greek yogurt, plain (11)	–	–
	Milk (31)	–	–

Food Group	Low GI (≤55)	Medium GI (56–69)	High GI (≥70)
Beans, Nuts & Legumes	Lentils (32) Chickpeas (28) Black Beans (30)	Black-eyed peas (58)	–
Snacks & Drinks	Popcorn (~55)	Light popcorn (65)	Pretzels (83)

1 Smart Real Life Strategies

Diabetes nutrition does not need to be complicated. The more realistic the plan is, the more likely you are to follow it.

Flavor Without Access Salt

Use herbs, spices, lemon or lime juice, garlic powder, onion powder, pepper blends, vinegar, and citrus zest to build flavor while protecting blood pressure.

Limit Added Sugars (Without Guilt)

The American Heart Association recommends limiting added sugars, which can[4]:

- Support blood sugar control
- Reduce craving
- Support heart and metabolic health by reducing inflammation in the body
- Help prevent weight gain and high triglycerides
- **Beverages**

Choose water and calorie-free beverages more often over sugary drinks and juice. Water helps to flush out sugar from the body.

Sweets

Enjoy sweets intentionally, not unexpectedly. You will find some dessert options in this cookbook.

FDA-Approved Sweeteners Are Considered Safe

Low-and no-calorie sweeteners that can help reduce added sugar intake include:

- Sucralose
- Aspartame
- Stevia
- Monk-Fruit

Food Label Reading

Know what to look for on food labels.

Focus on:

- Serving size
- Total carbohydrates
- Fiber
- Added sugars
- Protein
- Sodium

Nutrition Facts	
Approx. 14 servings per container	
Serving size 1 slice (48g)	
Amount per serving	
Calories	**100**
	% Daily Value*
Total Fat 0.5g	1%
Saturated Fat 0g	0%
Trans Fat 0g	
Cholesterol 0mg	0%
Sodium 115mg	5%
Total Carbohydrate 21g	7%
Dietary Fiber 4g	15%
Total Sugar 1g	
Includes 1g Added Sugars	2%
Protein 4g	
Vitamin D 0mcg	0%
Calcium 25mg	0%
Iron .7mg	4%
Potassium 60mg	0%

*The % Daily Value (DV) tells you how much a nutrient in a serving of food contributes to a daily diet. 2,000 calories a day is used for general nutrition advice.

Aim For:

- Higher fiber (greater than 3 g per serving)
- Moderate total carbs
- Some protein
- Lower added sugars (less than 5 grams added sugar or < 10% of DV)
- Lower sodium <140 mg per serving or less than 2300 mg per day.

Meal Planning That Works in Real Life

Meal planning doesn't have to mean complicated schedules, hours of prep work, or giving up spontaneity. It simply creates structure, and structure makes healthy eating easier, less stressful, and more affordable.

One of my clients, Gwen, learned this firsthand. She ate out for two of her three meals every day because she felt too busy and too tired to figure out meals at home. She wasn't trying to make unhealthy choices; she was doing the best she could with the time and energy she had. But the cost added up quickly, and her blood sugars stayed unpredictable.

During one appointment, she told me, "I know what I'm supposed to eat... I just never have it ready when I need it." That was her turning point. She didn't need a stricter diet; she needed a plan that worked with her life.

Together, we focused on something simple:

Spending just one hour on the weekend preparing for the week ahead.

Not cooking all the meals — just planning:

- 3–4 go-to dinners for the week
- Ingredients for easy breakfasts and lunches
- A couple of backup meal options for busy nights

Within a few weeks, Gwen wasn't eating out twice a day anymore. She felt calmer, spent less money, had fewer blood sugar spikes after meals, and actually enjoyed the food she was eating. She didn't become a different person; she just had a system that supported her.

The Takeaway

Meal planning isn't about perfection. It's about making healthy eating automatic instead of stressful.

Small steps can make a big difference:

- Reuse ingredients across multiple recipes
- Keep a few easy meals stocked for busy nights.
- Choose 5–7 reliable meals instead of starting from zero every week.
- Use the weekend to make choices your weekday self will appreciate.

Even One Intentional Hour A Week Can Lead To:

- Better blood sugar
- Less stress
- More confidence
- Lower grocery costs
- Less temptation to eat out by default

Meal planning isn't about restriction; it's about freedom. It frees up time, money, energy, and mental space while helping your body feel supported and steady.

Meal Planning that Works in Real Life

Meal planning does not have to be strict. A simple approach makes healthy eating more automatic:

- Choose 5–7 go-to meals
- Reuse ingredients across multiple mealsCook once and enjoy leftovers

the next day

- Keep backup meals for busy nights

Use affordable staples: eggs, tuna, frozen vegetables, beans, yogurt, oats, whole-grain pasta, and brown rice.

Meal Planning Reduces

- Grocery costs
- Food waste
- Stress around eating
- Last-minute, high-sugar or high-sodium choices

Consistency makes more difference than perfection.

You Can Do This

Managing diabetes is not about following rigid rules; it is about learning how to support your body, your energy, and your long-term health.

You don't have to change everything at once. Every balanced meal counts. Every thoughtful choice supports you.

With 60 easy recipes and meal plans, realistic ingredients, and practical guidance, this cookbook is here to help you:

- Feel confident about food choices
- Support your blood sugar and heart health
- Enjoy food without guilt
- Take care of your body in a way that works in your real life

Let's make healthy eating simple again. Let's take care of your body, one easy meal at a time.

Quick note:

If you want to truly understand why blood sugar spikes happen and how food, habits, and daily choices all connect...

We recommend our book The Diabetes Reset by Marianne Greene and Elizabeth Berkey.

It breaks diabetes down into clear, simple explanations so the confusion disappears and the full picture finally clicks. Many readers say it's the first time diabetes actually made sense.

You'll find the link at the end of this book, just before the resource section at the end of the book.

Don't forget your bonuses

These tools come in handy:

◊ Avoid Sugar Spikes – Carb Swap Cheat Sheet (PDF)
◊ DIY Meal Planner – make your own plan & adjust recipes (Printable PDF)
◊ 11 Tips for Staying Active Safely With Diabetes (PDF)
◊ Information about becoming an advance reader for our next book

The Bonus section is listed at the end of the Table of Contents

All bonuses are optional and waiting for you when you're ready.

Elizabeth Berkey, MS, RDN, LD, CDCES, BC-ADM

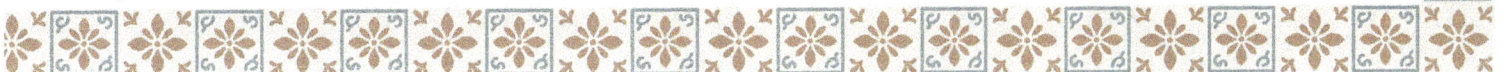

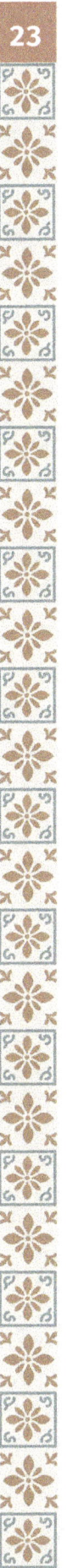

Day	Breakfast	Lunch	Dinner	Snacks
1	1 cup Protein Packed Peanut Butter Overnight Oats **p. 34** (38 g carb) with ½ Small Banana (11 g carb)	Fiesta Chicken Quesadilla (44 g carb) **p. 81** with 1 ½ cups Fresh Garden Green Salad **p. 65** (7 g carb) and 1-2 Tbsp. Light Dressing of choice	4-Tasty Teriyaki Turkey Meatballs (9 g carb) **p. 45** with 1 cup homestyle Garlic Mashed Potatoes with Skin **p. 56** (40g carb)& ½ cup Carrots **p. 68** (10g carb)	1 cup Creamy Greek Yogurt with Sugar-free Pudding (14 g carb) **p. 87**
2	2 Country Style Egg Bites **p. 36** (6 g carb) with 2 Slices of Whole-Grain Toast (30g carb) with 1-2 Tsp. of Light Margarine and 1-2 Mandarin Oranges (9-18 g carb).	1-Classic Tuna & Cheddar Melt **p. 82** (41 g carb) with 1 cup Raw Carrots (7 grams carb)	1-Quick Skillet Chicken Fajita (38 g carb) **p. 44** with 1 ½ cups Fresh Garden Green Salad (7 g carb) with 1-2 Tbsp. Light Dressing **p. 65**	10 oz. Smooth and Creamy Banana Berry Smoothie (14 g carbs) **p. 88**
3	1-Hearty Breakfast Burritos (39 g carb) **p. 35** with 1 cup of Berries (15 g carb)	1 cup Hearty Homestyle Vegetable Soup (41 g carb) **p. 83** with ½ Turkey and Swiss Sandwich on Wheat Bread (15 g) with 1 Tbsp. Light Mayo or Mustard.	1 cup Cozy Chicken Noodle Casserole (42g carb) **p. 46** with 1 ½ cups Fresh Green Garden Salad (7 g carb) with 1-2 Tbsp. Light Dressing. **p. 65**	1 mug cup -Warm Sugar-Free Brownie in a Mug (14 g carb) **p. 89**
4	1 Cheesy Black Bean Breakfast Quesadillas (42 g carb) **p. 38**	1 cup Old Fashioned Chicken Noodle Soup (31 g carb) **p. 84** and ½ Deli Low Sodium Chicken Sandwich on Whole-Wheat (15 g carb) with 1 Tbsp. Light Mayo or Mustard.	4 oz. Lemon Chicken (4 g carb) **p. 43** with 1 cup Parmesan Risotto (44 g carb) **p. 57** and 1 cup Roasted Asparagus with Lemon **p. 61** (7 g carb)	½ cup Creamy Sweet Strawberry Mousse (19 g carb) **p. 90**
5	1 ¼ cups Farmhouse Vegie Breakfast Scramble (20 g carb) **p. 37** with 2 slices of Rye Bread (30 g carb) and 1 Tbsp. Light Margarine.	2 cups Crisp Chicken Caesar Salad with Creamy Homemade Caesar Dressing **p. 85** (11 g carb), 1 slice Whole-Wheat Bread (15 g carb) with 1-2 Tsp. of Light Margarine and 1 cup of Mixed Fresh Fruit (15 g carb).	2 Quick and Crispy Salmon Patties (22 g carb **p. 48** with ½ cup Cozy Spinach-Parmesan Ozo Skillet (23 g carb), ½ cup Crispy Oven Roasted Summer Squash **p. 67** (4 g carb)	6 Whole-Grain Crackers (15 g carb) with Savory 2 Tbsp. Tuna Salad (3 g carb) **p. 93**

Day	Breakfast	Lunch	Dinner	Snacks
6	1 cup Creamy Berry Nut Crunch Yogurt Parfait **p. 40** (36 g carb) with ½ Toasted Whole-Wheat Mini Bagel (15g carb) with 1 Tbsp. Whipped Cream Cheese (1-2 g carb)	2 cups Greek Salad with Chickpeas & Feta (28 g carb) **p. 86** with 1 cup of mixed fruit (15 g carb)	1 cup Tuna Noodle Casserole (40 g carb **p. 49** with 1 ½ cups Fresh Green Salad (7 g carb) and 1-2 Tbsp. Light Dressing **p. 65**	2 Chewy Chocolate Banana Oat Cookies (32 g carb) **p. 91**
7	1 Crispy Turkey Bacon-Egg Quesadilla Melt (37 g carb) **p. 39** with 1 cup Mixed Berries (15 g carb)	1 cup Hearty Homestyle Vegetable Chili (47 g carb) **p. 73** with 1 Small Apple (15 g carb)	1 cup Homestyle Beef and Noodles **p. 51** (46 g carb) with 1 cup Oven Roasted Broccoli with Parmesan (11 g carb **p. 60**	½ cup Spiced Pumpkin Cream Cup (20 g carb) **p. 92**
8	1 ¼ cup Farmhouse Vegie Breakfast Scramble (20 g carb) **p. 37** with a Whole-Grain English Muffin (30 g) with 1 Tbsp. Light Margarine	2 cups Wholesome Turkey Nourish Bowl (37 g carb) **p. 53** with 1 Hard Boiled Egg and 1 Medium Orange (15 g carb)	1 Fillet (5 oz) Zesty Lemon Pepper Tilapia **p. 54** (4 g carb) with 1 cup Zesty Roasted Asparagus with Lemon (7 g carb) **p. 61** and 1 cup Hearty Wild Rice Pilaf (44 g carb) **p. 59**	1 cup Creamy Greek Yogurt with Sugar-Free Pudding (14 g carb) **p. 87**
9	1 cup Creamy Berry Nut Crunch Yogurt Parfait (36 g carb) **p. 40** with 1 slice of Whole-Grain toast (15 g carb) with 1-2 Tbsp. Natural Peanut Butter	1-Cozy Black Bean & Corn Quesadillas (32 g carb) **p. 72** with 1 ½ cups Fresh Green Garden Salad (7 g carb), and 1-2 Tbsp. Light Dressing of choice. **p. 65**	4 oz. Quick and Easy Creamy Garlic Pork Chops (8 g carb) **p. 55** with 1 cup Homestyle Garlic Mashed Potatoes with Skin (40 g carb) **p. 56** and ½ cup Savory Garlic Sauteed Mushrooms (6 g carb) **p. 66**	10 oz. Smooth and Creamy Banana Berry Smoothie (14 g carb) **p. 88**
10	1-Crispy Turkey Bacon–Egg Quesadilla Melt (37 g) **p. 39** with ¼ cup Salsa (4 g carb) and 1 cup Canteloupe (15 g carb)	1 ¼ cup Sweet Savory Teriyaki Edamame Noodle Bowl (56 g carb) **p. 76**	1 ¼ cup Hearty Veggie Enchilada Bake **p. 74** (47 g carb) with ½ cup of Mixed Fruit (9 g carb)	1 mug cake- Warm Sugar-Free Brownie in a Mug (14 g carb) **p. 89**

Day	Breakfast	Lunch	Dinner	Snacks
11	1 Homestyle Oat Breakfast Bar (39 g) **p. 42** and 2 Cutie Tangerines (15 g carb)	1 Fiesta Chicken Quesadilla (38 g carb) **p. 81** with ¼ cup Salsa (4 g carb) and 1 Tbsp. Light Sour Cream (1 g carb) and a small Apple (15 g carb)	1 ¼ cup Creamy Parmesan Zucchini Carbonara (53 g carb) **p. 79** with 1 ½ cups Fresh Green Garden Salad (7 g carb) with 1-2 Tbsp. Light Dressing of choice. **p. 65**	1 cup Creamy Greek Yogurt with Sugar-Free Pudding (14 g carb) **p. 87**
12	1-Hearty Fruit & Fiber Muffin (36 g carb) **p. 41** with 2 Egg Bites (6 g carb) **p. 36**	1 Classic Tuna and Cheddar Melt (41 g carb) **p. 82** with 1 Medium Fresh Peach (15 g carb)	1 ¼ cup Sweet Savory Teriyaki Edamame Noodle Bowl (56 g carb) **p. 76**	½ cup Creamy Sweet Strawberry Mousse (19 g carb) **p. 90** with 1 Tbsp. Crushed Graham Crackers (5 g carb)
13	2 cups Avocado Egg Protein Power Bowl (29 g carb) **p. 43** and 17 Small Grapes (15 g carb)	1 cup Hearty Homestyle Vegetable Soup (41 g carb) **p. 83** with ½ Deli Chicken and Cheddar Cheese Sandwich on Whole-Wheat Bread (15 g carb) with 1-2 Tbsp. Light Mayo.	4 Tasty Teriyaki Turkey Meatballs (9 g carb) **p. 45** with 1 cup Savory Brown Rice Pilaf (44 g carb) **p. 58** and ½ cup Steamed Broccoli (5 g carb) **p. 60**	½ cup Spiced Pumpkin Cream Cup (20 g carb) **p. 92** with 1 Tbsp. of Chopped Pecans (1 g carb)
14	1 cup Protein Packed Peanut Butter Overnight Oats (38 g carb) **p. 34** with ¼ cup Blueberries (5 g carb) and 1 Tbsp. Ground Flax Seed (2 g carb)	1 cup Old-Fashioned Chicken Noodle Soup (31 g carb) **p. 84** with ½ Deli Turkey and Swiss Sandwich on Whole-Grain Bread (15 g carb) with 1 Tbsp. Light Mayo and 1/2 cup Mixed Berries (9 g carb)	1 cup Cozy Chicken Noodle Casserole (42 g carb) **p. 46**, ½ cup Strawberries (6 g carb) with 1 ½ cup Fresh Garden Green Salad (7 g carb) with 1-2 Tbsp. Light Dressing of choice. **p. 65**	6 Whole-Grain Crackers (15 g carb) with 2 Tbsp. Savory Tuna Salad (3 g carb) **p. 93**
15	2 cups Avocado Egg Protein Power Bowl (29 g carb) **p. 43** with 1 Small Banana (30 g carb)	2 cups Crisp Chicken Caesar Salad with Creamy Homemade Caesar Dressing (11 g carb) **p. 85** with ½ Turkey and Swiss Sandwich on Whole-Wheat Bread (15 g carb) with 1 Tbsp. Light Mayo or Mustard and 1 ¼ cup Strawberries (15 g carb)	4 oz. Zesty Lemon Chicken (4 g carb) **p. 47** with ½ cup Creamy Cheesy Broccoli Couscous (21 g carb) **p. 70** and 1 cup Roasted Green Beans with Tomatoes (12 g carb) **p. 62** and ½ cup Canned Peaches in Water (15 g carb)	¼ cup Homestyle Hummus with 1 cup Fresh Veggies (27 g carb) **p. 94**

Day	Breakfast	Lunch	Dinner	Snacks
16	2 Country-Style Egg Bites (6 g carb) **p. 36** with 2 slices Whole-Grain Toast (30 g carb), 1 with 1-2 Tsp. of Light Margarine and 2 Cutie Tangerines (15 g carb)	2 cups Hearty Greek Salad with Chickpeas & Feta (28 g carb) with 1 Small Orange (15 g carb) **p. 86**	4 Rustic Toasted Ravioli and ½ cup Veggies (48 g carb) **p. 71** with ½ cup of Mixed Fruit (9 g carb)	2 Easy Turkey & Cheddar Roll-Ups (7 g carb) **p. 95** with 6 Triscuits (20 g carb)
17	1 Hearty Breakfast Burritos (39 g carb) **p. 35** with ½ of a Mango (15 g carb)	2 cups Wholesome Turkey Nourish Bowl (37 g carb) **p. 53** with ½ cup of Canned Pears in water (15 g carb)	2 Quick and Crispy Salmon Patties (22 g carb) **p. 48** with ½ cup Whole-Grain Orzo with Spinach & Parmesan (23 g carb) **p. 69** and ½ cup Roasted Zucchini & Summer Squash (4 g carb)	2 cups Sweet & Salty Protein Popcorn (23 g carb) **p. 96**
18	1 Cheesy Black Bean Breakfast Quesadillas (42 g carb)**p. 38** with 2 Small Plums (14 g carb)	1 cup Hearty Homestyle Vegetable Chili (47 g carb) **p. 73** with 5 Whole-Grain Saltines (12 g carb)	1 cup Creamy Tuna Noodle Casserole (40 g carb) **p. 49** with ¾ cup Fresh Pineapple (15 g carb)	10 oz. Smooth and Creamy Banana Berry Smoothie (14 g carb) **p. 88**
19	1 ¼ cup Farmhouse Vegie Breakfast Scramble (20 g carb) **p. 37** with Mini Whole Grain Bagel (30 g carb) with 1-2 Tbsp. Whipped Cream Cheese (1 g carb).	1 Cozy Black Bean & Corn Quesadillas (32 g carb) with 1 cup of Papaya (15 g carb) **p. 72**	1 cup Homestyle Beef and Noodles (46 g carb) **p. 51** with 1 cup Oven Roasted Broccoli with Parmesan (11 g carb) **p. 60**	1 mug cake-Warm Sugar-Free Brownie in a Mug (14 g carb) **p. 89**
20	1 cup Creamy Berry Nut Crunch Yogurt Parfait (36 g carb) **p. 40** with 1 Slice of Sourdough Toast (15 g carb) with 1-2 Tsp. Light Margarine.	1 Fiesta Chicken Quesadilla (38 g carb) with 1 Small Apple (15 g carb) **p. 81**	1 ¼ cup Hearty Veggie Enchilada Bake (47 carb) **p. 74** with 1 cup of Watermelon (11 g carb)	½ cup Creamy Sweet Strawberry Mousse (19 g carb) **p. 90**
	1 Crispy Turkey Bacon-Egg Quesadilla Melt (37 g carb) **p. 39** with 1 Small Orange (15 g carb)	1 Classic Tuna and Cheddar Melt (41 g carb) **p. 82** with 1 Small Apple (15 g carb)	4 oz. Quick and Easy Creamy Garlic Pork Chops (8 g carb) **p. 55** with 1 ¼ cup Cozy Edamame Rice Skillet (22 g carb) **p. 77** and ½ cup Unsweetened Apple sauce (15 g carb)	2 Chewy Chocolate Banana Oat Cookies (32 g carb) **p. 91**

Day	Breakfast	Lunch	Dinner	Snacks
22	1 ¼ cup Farmhouse Vegie Breakfast Scramble (20 g carb) **p. 37** with 1 cup of Fresh Berries (15 g carb)	1 cup Hearty Homestyle Vegetable Soup (41 g carb) **p. 83** with 1 Slice of Sourdough Bread (15 g carb) with 1-2 Tsp. of Light Margarine	4 Tasty Teriyaki Turkey Meatballs (9 g carb) **p. 45** with 1 cup Crispy Oven Roasted Sweet Potatoes (27 g carb) **p. 64** and ½ cup Savory Sauteed Mushrooms (6 g carb) **p. 66**	½ cup Spiced Pumpkin Cream Cup (20 g carb) **p. 92**
23	1 cup Creamy Berry Nut Crunch Yogurt Parfait (36 g carb) **p. 40** with 2 Egg Bites (6 g carb) **p. 36**	1 cup Old Fashioned Chicken Noodle Soup (31 g carb) **p. 84** with 5 Whole-Grain Saltines (12 g carb) with 1 Cutie Tangerine (8 g carb)	4 oz. Zesty Lemon Chicken (4 g carb) **p. 47** with 6 Country Oven Roasted Cauliflower Steaks (11 g carb) **p. 63** with ½ cup Creamy Cheesy Broccoli Couscous (21 g carb) **p. 70**	6 Whole-Grain Crackers (15 g carb) with 2 Tbsp. Savory Tuna Salad (3 g carb) **p. 93**
24	1 Crispy Turkey Bacon–Egg Quesadilla Melt (37 g carb) **p. 39** with 1 cup Honey Dew Melon (15 g carb)	2 cups Crisp Chicken Caesar Salad with Creamy Homemade Caesar Dressing (11 g carb) **p. 85** with 1 cup mixed Fruit (15 g carb) and 1 Slice of Sourdough Bread (15 g carb) with 1-2 Tsp. of Light Margarine	1 cup Cozy Chicken Noodle Casserole (42 g carb) with 17 Small Grapes (15 g carb) **p. 46**	¼ cup Homestyle Hummus with 1 cup Fresh Veggies (27 g carb) **p. 94**
25	1 Homestyle Oat Breakfast Bars (39 g carb) with ¾ cup Greek Yogurt (8 g carb) **p. 42**	2 cup Hearty Greek Salad with Chickpeas & Feta (28 g carb) **p. 86** with ½ Whole-Grain Pita (15 g carb)	2 Quick and Crispy Salmon Patties (22 g carb) **p. 48** with ½ cup Cozy Spinach Parmesan Orzo (23 g carb) **p. 69** and 1 ½ cups Fresh Garden Green Salad (11 g carb) **p. 65** with 1-2 Tbsp. of Light Dressing	2 Easy Turkey & Cheddar Roll-Ups (7 g carb) with 1 Clementine (15 g carb) **p. 95**
26	1 Hearty Fruit & Fiber Muffins (36 g carb) **p. 41** with 1 Hard Boiled Egg	1 Fiesta Chicken Quesadilla (38 g carb) **p. 81** with ¾ cup Fresh Pineapple (15 g carb)	1 cup Creamy Tuna Noodle Casserole (40 g carb) **p. 49** with 1 cup Fresh Berries (15 g carb)	2 cups Sweet & Salty Protein Popcorn (23 g carb) **p. 96**
27	2 cups Avocado Egg Protein Power Bowl (29 g carb) **p. 43** plus 1 Small Banana (30 g carb)	1 Classic Tuna and Cheddar Melt (41 g carb) **p. 82** with 1 Small Apple (15 g carb)	4 oz. Quick and Easy Creamy Garlic Pork Chops (8 g carb) **p. 55** with 1 cup Creamy Parmesan Risotto (44 g carb)	1 cup Creamy Greek Yogurt with Sugar-Free Pudding (14 g carb) **p. 87** and a Few Blueberries
28	1 cup Protein Packed Peanut Butter Overnight Oats (38 g carb) **p. 34** with 1 Hard Boiled Egg	1 cup Hearty Homestyle Vegetable Soup (41 g carb) **p. 83** with ½ Deli Turkey and Provolone Sandwich (15 g carb) with 1 Tbsp. Light Mayo	1 cup Homestyle Beef and Noodles (46 g carb) **p. 51** with 1 cup Oven Roasted Broccoli with Parmesan (11 g carb) **p. 60**	10 oz. Smooth and Creamy Banana Berry Smoothie (14 g carb) **p. 88**

60 DAY MEAL PLAN - MONTH 2

Day	Breakfast	Lunch	Dinner	Snacks
1	2-Country Style Egg Bites (6 g carb) **p. 36** with 2 slices of Whole-Grain Toast (30 g carb) with 1-2 Tsp. of Light Margarine and 1 cup Mixed Berries (15 g carb)	1 cup Old Fashioned Chicken Noodle Soup (31 g carb) **p. 84** with 6 Whole-Grain Saltine Crackers (15 g carb)	2 cups Wholesome Turkey Nourish Bowl (37 g carb) **p. 53** with 1 cup of Melon (15 g carb)	1 mug cake- Warm Sugar- Free Brownie in a Mug (14 g carb) **p. 89** with a Few Raspberries
2	2-Country Style Egg Bites (6 g carb) **p. 36** with 2 slices of Whole-Grain Toast (30 g carb) with 1-2 Tsp. of Light Margarine and 1 cup Mixed Berries (15 g carb)	1 ½ cup Crisp Chicken Caesar Salad with Creamy Homemade Caesar Dressing (11 g carb) **p. 85** with 1 Large Apple (30 g carb)	1 Fillet (5 oz.) Zesty Lemon Pepper Tilapia (4 g carb) **p. 54** with 1 cup Hearty Wild Rice (44 g carb) **p. 59** and 1 cup Zesty Roasted Asparagus with Lemon (7 g carb)**p. 61**	1/ 2 cup Creamy Sweet Strawberry Mousse (19 g carb)**p. 90**
3	1 Cheesy Black Bean Breakfast Quesadillas (42 g carb) **p. 38** with 1 Medium Peach (15 g carb)	2 cups Hearty Greek Salad with Chickpeas & Feta (28 g carb) **p. 86** and 12 Whole-Grain Pita Chips (15 g)	4 Tasty Teriyaki Turkey Meatballs (9 g carb) **p. 45** with 1 cup Homestyle Garlic Mashed Potatoes with Skin (40 g carb) **p. 56** and ½ cup Carmelized Oven Roasted Carrots (10 g Carb) **p. 68**	2 Chewy Chocolate Banana Oat Cookies (27 g carb) **p. 91**
4	1 ¼ cup Farmhouse Vegie Breakfast Scramble (20 g carb) **p. 37** with 8-inch Whole Grain Tortilla (25 g carb)	2 cups Wholesome Turkey Nourish Bowl (37 g carb) **p. 53** with 1 cup of Mixed Fruit (15 g carb)	4 oz Quick and Easy Creamy Garlic Pork Chops (8 g carb) **p. 55** with 1 cup Roasted Green Beans & Tomatoes (12 g carb) **p.62** and 1 cup Homestyle Garlic Mashed Potatoes with Skin (40 g carb) **p. 56**	½ cup Spiced Pumpkin Cream Cup (20 g carb) **p. 92** with 1 Tbsp. Whipped Cream
5	1 cup Creamy Berry Nut Crunch Yogurt Parfait (36 g carb) **p. 40** with 2 Egg Bites (6 g carb) **p. 36**	1 cup Hearty Homestyle Vegetable Chili (47 g carb) **p. 73** with 5 Whole-Grain Tortilla Chips (12 g carb)	1 Quick Skillet Chicken Fajitas (38 g carb) **p. 44** with ½ cup Unsweetened Apple Sauce (15 g carb)	6 Whole-Grain Crackers (15 g carb) with 2 Tbsp. Savory Tuna Salad (3 g carb) **p. 93**

Day	Breakfast	Lunch	Dinner	Snacks
6	1 Crispy Turkey Bacon–Egg Quesadilla Melt (37 g carb) **p. 39** with 1 cup Melon (15 g carb)	1 Classic Tuna and Ceddar Melt (41 g carb) **p. 82** with 1 Small Apple (15 g carb)	1 ¼ cup Buttery Soy-Garlic Linguine with Mushrooms **p. 66** & Edamame (49 g carb) **p. 78**	¼ cup Homestyle Hummus with 1 cup Fresh Veggies (27 g carb) **p.94**
7	1 Homestyle Oat Breakfast Bars (39 g carb) **p. 42** with ¾ cup Greek Yogurt (8 g carb)	1 ¼ cup Sweet Savory Teriyaki Edamame Noodle Bowl (56 g carb) **p. 76**	1 cup Cozy Chicken Noodle Casserole (42 g carb) **p. 46** with 1 cup Mixed Fruit (15 g carb)	2 Easy Turkey & Cheddar Roll-Ups (7 g carb) **p. 95** with 17 Small Grapes (15 g carb)
8	1 Hearty Fruit & Fiber Muffin (36 g carb) **p. 41** with 1 cup Mixed Berries (15 g carb)	1 Cozy Black Bean & Corn Quesadillas (32 g carb) **p. 72** with ¼ cup Salsa (6 g carb) and 2 Tbsp. Light Sour Cream (2 g carb)	4 oz. Zesty Lemon Chicken (4 g carb) **p. 47** with 1 cup Crispy Oven Roasted Sweet Potatos (27 g carb) **p. 64** and 6 County Oven Roasted Cauliflower Steaks (11 g carb) **p. 63**	2 cup Sweet & Salty Protein Popcorn (23 g carb) **p. 96**
9	2 cups Avocado Egg Protein Power Bowl (29 g carb) **p. 43** with 1 Small Orange (15 g carb)	1 Fiesta Chicken Quesadilla (44 g carb) **p. 81** with ¼ cup Salsa (6 g carb) and 2 Tbsp. Light Sour Cream (2 g carb)	2 Quick and Crispy Salmon Patties (37 g carb) **p. 48** with ½ cup Carmelized Oven Roasted Carrots (10 g carb) **p. 68** and 1 ½ cups Fresh Garden Green Salad (7 g carb) **p. 65** with Choice of 1-2 Tbsp. of Light Dressing	½ cup Creamy Greek Yogurt with Sugar-Free Pudding (14 g carb) **p. 87**
10	2 Country Style Egg Bites (6 g carb) **p. 36** with 1 Whole-Grain Mini Bagel (30 g carb) and 2 Tbsp. Whipped Cream Cheese (2 g carb)	1 cup Hearty Homestyle Vegetable Chili (47 g carb) **p. 73** with 2 Tbsp. Light Sour Cream (2 g carb), ¼ cup Cheddar Cheese (2 g carb), and 1 Slice of Whole-Grain Bread (15 g carb) with 1-2 Tsp. Light Margarine	1 ¼ cup Creamy Parmesan Zucchini Carbonara (53 g carb) **p. 79**	10 oz. Smooth and Creamy Banana Berry Smoothie (14 g carb) **p. 88**
11	1 Hearty Breakfast Burritos (39 g carb) with 1 cup of Mixed Fruit (15 g carb) **p. 35**	2 cups Savory Edamame Nourish Bowl (46 g carb) **p. 78**	1 cup Homestyle Beef and Noodles (46 g carb) **p. 51** with 1 cup Roasted Green Beans & Tomatoes (12 g carb) **p. 62**	1 mug cake-Warm Sugar-Free Brownie in a Mug (14 g carb) **p. 89**

Day	Breakfast	Lunch	Dinner	Snacks
12	1 cup Protein Packed Peanut Butter Overnight Oats (38 carb) **p. 34** with ½ Small Banana (15 g carb)	1 Classic Tuna and Cheddar Melt (41 g carb) **p. 82** with 1 cup of Raw Carrots (6 g carb)	4 Rustic Toasted Ravioli and ½ cup Veggies (48 g carb) **p. 71** with 1 Small Plum (8 g carb)	½ cup Creamy Sweet Strawberry Mousse (19 g carb) **p. 90**
13	1 ¼ cup Farmhouse Vegie Breakfast Scramble (20 g carb) **p. 37** with 2 Slices Rye Toast (30 g carb) with 1-2 Tbsp. Light Margarine	1 cup Hearty Homestyle Vegetable Soup (41 g carb) **p. 83** with a Few Oyster Crackers and 1 small Apple (15 g carb)	1 ¼ cup Cozy Edamame Rice Skillet (22 g carb) **p. 77** with 12 Fresh Cherries (15 g carb)	1 Chewy Chocolate Banana Oat Cookies (32 g carb) **p. 91**
14	1 cup Creamy Berry Nut Crunch Yogurt Parfait (36 g carb) **p. 40** with 2 Egg Bites (6 g carb) **p. 36**	1 cup Old Fashioned Chicken Noodle Soup (31 g carb) **p. 84** with ½ Deli Turkey and Baby Swiss Sandwich on 9-grain Bread (15 g carb) with 1 Tbsp. Light Mayo or Mustard	2-Quick and Crispy Salmon Patties (37 g carb) **p. 48** with 3 oz. Baked Potato (15 g carb) with 1 Tbsp. Light Margarine and 1 ½ cupa Fresh Garden Green Salad (7 g carb) with 1-2 Tbsp. Light Dressing of Choice **p. 65**	½ cup Spiced Pumpkin Cream Cup (20 g carb) **p. 92**
15	1 Crispy Turkey Bacon–Egg Quesadilla Melt (37 g carb) **p. 39** with ½ cup Canned Pears (15 g carb)	2 cups Crisp Chicken Caesar Salad with Creamy Homemade Caesar Dressing (11 g carb) **p. 85** with 6 Whole-Grain Crackers (15 g Carb) and 2 Cutie Tangerines (15 g carb)	2 cups Wholesome Turkey Nourish Bowl (37 g carb) **p. 53** with 1 cup of Mixed Fruit (15 g carb)	6 Whole-Grain Crackers (15 g carb) with 2 Tbsp. Savory Tuna Salad (3 g carb) **p. 93**
16	1 Homestyle Oat Breakfast Bar (39 g carb) **p. 42** with 1 Hard Boiled Egg and ½ cup of Mixed Fruit (8 g carb)	2 cups Hearty Greek Salad with Chickpeas & Feta (28 g carb) **p. 86** with ½ a Whole-Grain Pita Bread (15 g carb)	1 cup Homestyle Beef and Noodles (46 g carb) **p. 51** with 1 cup Oven Roasted Broccoli with Parmesan (11 g carb) **p. 60**	1 cup Creamy Greek Yogurt with Sugar-Free Pudding (14 g carb) **p. 87**
17	1 Hearty Fruit & Fiber Muffin (36 g carb) **p. 41** with 1 cup of Canteloupe (15 g carb)	1 Fiesta Chicken Quesadilla (44 g carb) **p. 81** with 1 Small Apple (15 g carb)	4 oz. Quick and Easy Creamy Garlic Pork Chops (8 g carb) **p. 55** with 1 cup Crispy Oven Roasted Sweet Potatoes (27 g carb) **p. 64** and ½ cup Savory Garlic Sautéed Mushrooms (6 g carb) **p. 66**	10 oz. Smooth and Creamy Banana Berry Smoothie (14 g carb) **p. 88**

Day	Breakfast	Lunch	Dinner	Snacks
18	2 cups Avocado Egg Protein Power Bowl (29 g carb) **p. 43** with 1 cup Mixed Fruit (15 g carb)	1 Classic Tuna and Cheddar Melt (41 g carb) **p. 82** with 1 Small Orange (15 g carb)	1 cup Hearty Homestyle Vegetable Chili (47 g carb) **p. 73** with ½ Roast Beef and Cheddar Sandwich on Whole-Wheat Bread (15 g carb)	1 mug cake-Warm Sugar-Free Brownie in a Mug (14 g carb) **p. 89**
19	1 cup Protein Packed Peanut Butter Overnight Oats (38 g carb) **p. 34** with ½ Banana (15 g carb) and 1 Hard Boiled Egg	1 cup Hearty Homestyle Vegetable Soup (41 g carb) **p. 83** with ½ Low Sodium Ham and Cheese Sandwich (15 g carb) with 1-2 Tsp. Light Mayo	4 Rustic Toasted Ravioli and ½ cup Veggies (48 g carb) **p. 71** with 1 ½ cup Fresh Garden Green Salad (7 g carb) and 1-2 Tbsp. Light Dressing of Choice **p. 65**	½ cup Creamy Sweet Strawberry Mousse (19 g carb) with 1 Tbsp. Whipped Cream **p. 90**
20	2 Country Style Egg Bites (6 g carb) **p. 36** with 1 Whole-Grain English Muffin (30 g carb) with 1-2 Tsp. Light Margarine	1 cup Old Fashioned Chicken Noodle Soup (31 g carb) **p. 84** with ½ Tuna Fish Sandwich on Sourdough (18 g carb)	1 Cozy Black Bean & Corn Quesadillas (48 g carb) **p. 72** with 1 cup Mixed Berries (15 g carb)	2 Chewy Chocolate Banana Oat Cookies (27 g carb) **p. 91**
21	1 Hearty Breakfast Burrito (32 g carb) **p. 35** with 1 cup of Melon (15 g carb)	2 cups Crisp Chicken Caesar Salad with Creamy Homemade Caesar Dressing (11 g carb) **p. 85** and ½ cup Croutons (7 g carb) with 1 ¼ cups Strawberries (15 g carb)	4 Tasty Teriyaki Turkey Meatballs (9 g carb) **p. 45** with 1 cup Savory Brown Rice Pilaf (38 g carb) **p. 58** and 1 cup Sliced Strawberries (15 g carb)	½ cup Spiced Pumpkin Cream Cup (20 g carb) **p. 92** with 1 Tbsp. Whipped Cream
22	1 Cheesy Black Bean Breakfast Quesadillas (42 g carb) **p. 38** with 2 Plums (14 g carb)	2 cups Hearty Greek Salad with Chickpeas & Feta (28 g carb) **p. 86** with 12 Pita Chips (20 g carb) with 1 Cutie Tangerine (7 g carb)	1 cup Cozy Chicken Noodle Casserole (42 g carb) **p. 46** with ½ cup Fruit Cocktail (15 g carb)	6 Whole-Grain Crackers (15 g carb) with 2 Tbsp. Savory Tuna Salad (3 g carb) **p. 93**
23	1 ¼ cup Farmhouse Vegie Breakfast Scramble (20 g carb) **p. 37** with 2 Slices of Rye Toast (30 g carb) with 1-2 Tbsp. Light Margarine	1 cup Hearty Homestyle Vegetable Chili (47 g carb) **p. 73** with 5 Whole Grain Saltines (12 g carb) and ¼ cup of Cheddar Cheese	1 Quick Skillet Chicken Fajitas (38 g carb) **p. 44** with 1 ½ cup Fresh Garden Green Salad (7 g carb) **p. 65** with 1-2 Tbsp. Balsamic Vinegar Dressing	¼ cup Homestyle Hummus with 1 cup Fresh Veggies (27 g carb) **p. 94**

Day	Breakfast	Lunch	Dinner	Snacks
24	1 cup Creamy Berry Nut Crunch Yogurt Parfait (36 g carb) **p. 40** with 1 Hard Boiled Egg	1 ¼ cup Sweet Savory Teriyaki Edamame Noodle Bowl (56 g carb) **p. 76** with 1 ½ cups Fresh Garden Green Salad (7 g carb) with 1-2 Tbsp. of Light Dressing **p. 65**	1 Fillet (5 oz). Zesty Lemon Pepper Tilapia (4 g carb) **p. 54** with 1 cup Hearty Wild Rice Pilaf (44 g carb) **p. 59** and ½ cup Crispy Oven Roasted Summer Squash (4 g carb) **p. 67**	2 Easy Turkey & Cheddar Roll-Ups (7 g carb) **p. 95** with 2 Cutie Tangerines (15 g carb)
25	1 Crispy Turkey Bacon–Egg Quesadilla Melt (37 g carb) **p. 39** with ¾ cup Greek Yogurt (8 g carb)	1 ¼ cup Savory Edamame Nourish Bowl (46 g carb) **p. 78** with ½ cup Mixed Fruit (8 g carb)	1 ¼ cup Creamy Parmesan Zucchini Carbonara (53 g carb) **p. 79** with 1 ½ cup Fresh Garden Green Salad (7 g carb) with 1-2 Tbsp. of Light Dressing **p. 65**	2 cups Sweet & Salty Protein Popcorn (23 g carb) **p. 96**
26	1 cup Protein Packed Peanut Butter Overnight Oats (38 g carb) **p. 34** with 1 Small Apple (15 g carb)	1 Fiesta Chicken Quesadilla (44 g carb) **p. 81** with 17 small Grapes (15 g carb)	1 ¼ cup Buttery Soy-Garlic Linguine with Mushrooms & Edamame (49 g carb) **p. 80** with a 1 ½ cup Fresh Garden Green Salad with 1-2 Tbsp. Light Dressing of Choice **p. 65**	1 cup Creamy Greek Yogurt with Sugar-Free Pudding (14 g carb) **p. 87**
27	1 Hearty Fruit & Fiber Muffin (36 g carb) **p. 41** with 1 Hard-Boiled Egg	1 Classic Tuna and Cheddar Melt (41 g carb) **p. 82** with 1 cup Raspberries (15 g carb)	1 Quick Skillet Chicken Fajitas (38 g carb) **p. 44** with ½ cup Canned Pears (15 g carb)	10 oz. Smooth and Creamy Banana Berry Smoothie (14 g carb) **p. 88**
28	2 cups Avocado Egg Protein Power Bowl (29 g carb) **p. 43** with 1 cup Mixed Fruit (15 g carb)	1 cup Hearty Homestyle Vegetable Soup (41 g carb) with 6 Whole-Grain Crackers (15 g carb) **p. 83**	4 Tasty Teriyaki Turkey Meatballs (9 g carb) **p. 45** with 1 cup Homestyle Garlic Mashed Potatoes with Skin (40 g carb) **p. 56** and 1 cup Zesty Roasted Asparagus with Lemon (11 g carb) **p. 61**	1 mug cake-Warm Sugar-Free Brownie in a Mug (14 g carb) **p. 89**

How helpful is this book to you?

I'd love to hear what you think.

I personally read every review, and your feedback means the world to me.It only takes 30 seconds to leave a reivew.

It truly makes a huge difference for a small author like me—and it helps other Diabetes warriors discover this book too.

Here's how you can leave a review for the paperback:

- **Option 1: Scan the QR code to go straight to the review page.**

- **Option 2: Go to your Amazon orders, find this book, and click "Write a product review."**
- **Option 3: Search for the book title on Amazon, scroll down to the "Customer Reviews" section, and click "Write a Review."**

Once you're there, choose a star rating, a quick story about your experience, and submit!

Thank you so much. // MARIANNE <3

Protein-Packed Peanut Butter Overnight Oats

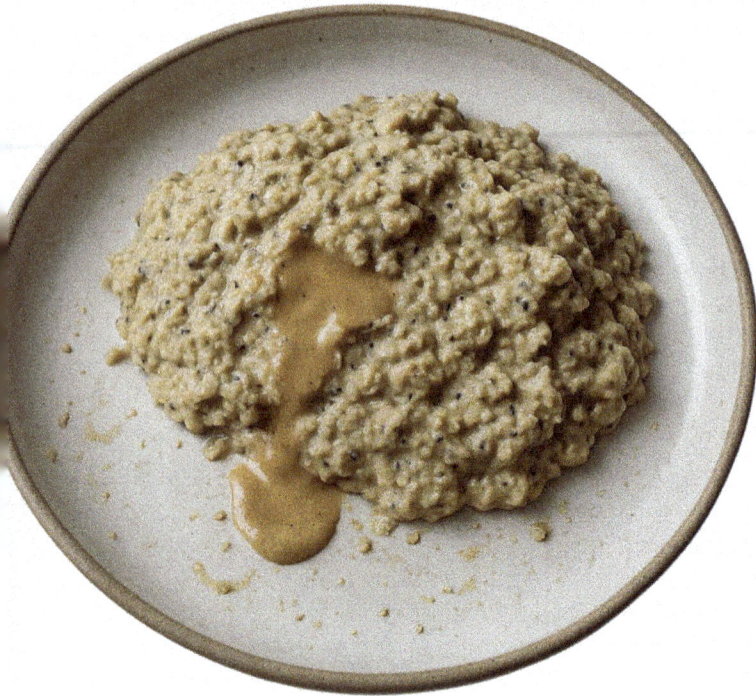

About this Recipe
Born for busy mornings, this creamy peanut butter oatmeal delivers lasting energy, keeps you full, supports muscles, and promotes gut health.

INGREDIENTS

2 cups old-fashioned oats
 • **2 cups unsweetened almond milk**
 • **½ cup powdered peanut butter (PB2 or similar)**
 • **¼ cup chia seeds**
 • **2 tbsp sugar-free maple syrup**
Optional seasonings: cinnamon, vanilla extract

Cook time
0'

Prep Time
5'

Servings
4x1cups

COST PER RECIPE
$9

GL
22/ HIGH

DIRECTIONS

1. **Add oats, almond milk, powdered peanut butter, chia seeds, and sugar-free syrup to a mixing bowl.**
2. **Stir well until evenly combined.**
3. **Divide into 4 containers or jars (1 cup each).**
4. **Refrigerate overnight or at least 6 hours.**
5. **Stir before serving. Add optional cinnamon or vanilla if desired.**

NUTRITION
Calories: 378 kcal | Protein: 38 g | Fat: 9 g | Carbohydrates: 38 g | Fiber: 8 g | Sodium: 356 mg

Creativity TWIST: Add ginger or Add ½ banana slices and a dash of cinnamon before serving for a comfort-food vibe (+8 g carbs), or mix in 2 tbsp low-fat Greek yogurt for extra creaminess and protein without increasing GL.

Hearty Breakfast Burritos

About this Recipe
Inspired by hearty morning traditions, these savory burritos deliver satisfying flavor, lasting fullness, and steady energy.

INGREDIENTS

- 4 whole-wheat tortillas
- 6 large eggs
- 1 cup reduced-fat shredded cheddar
- 1 cup diced bell peppers (fresh or frozen)
- 6 oz cooked lean turkey or chicken strips (diced)

Optional seasonings (not counted): black pepper, garlic powder, onion powder, salsa (1 tbsp is fine for flavor)

DIRECTIONS

1. Spray a skillet with cooking spray and heat over medium.
2. Add bell peppers and optional garlic powder, sauté 3 minutes.
3. Add eggs and scramble until fully cooked.
4. Stir in cooked turkey/chicken + cheddar until melted.
5. Divide the mixture evenly among 4 tortillas and roll burrito-style.
6. Serve warm or wrap individually for meal prep.

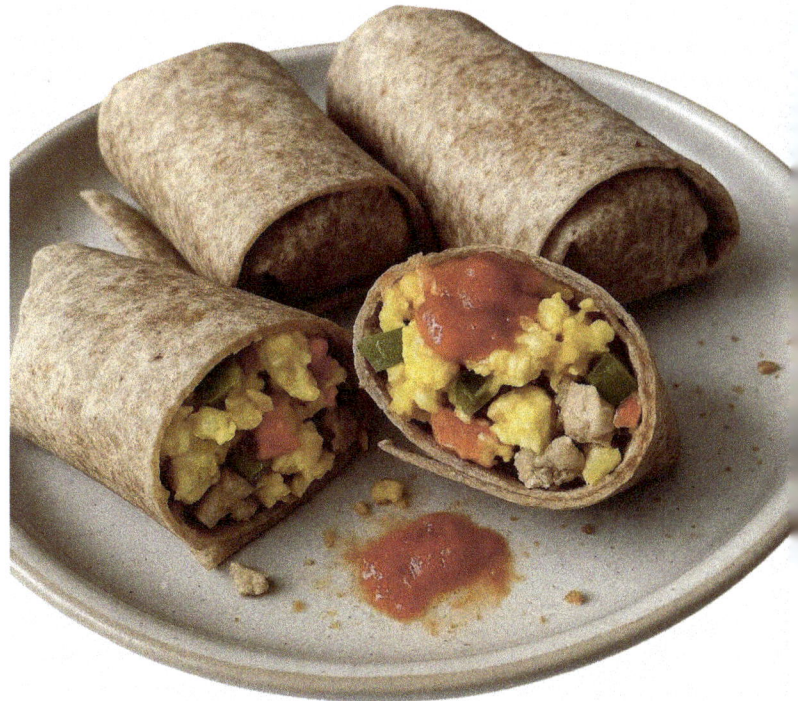

Servings 4 | Prep Time 10' | Cook time 10'

GL 15/ MID | COST PER RECIPE $9

NUTRITION (1 burrito per serving)
Calories: 412 kcal | Protein: 32 g | Fat: 9 g | Carbohydrates: 39 g | Fiber: 6 g | Sodium: 312 mg

Creativity TWIST: Swap turkey/chicken for black beans to create a vegetarian version with nearly the same calories and protein (from beans + cheddar). Can also add a dash of salsa without significantly increasing sodium.

Country Style Egg Bites

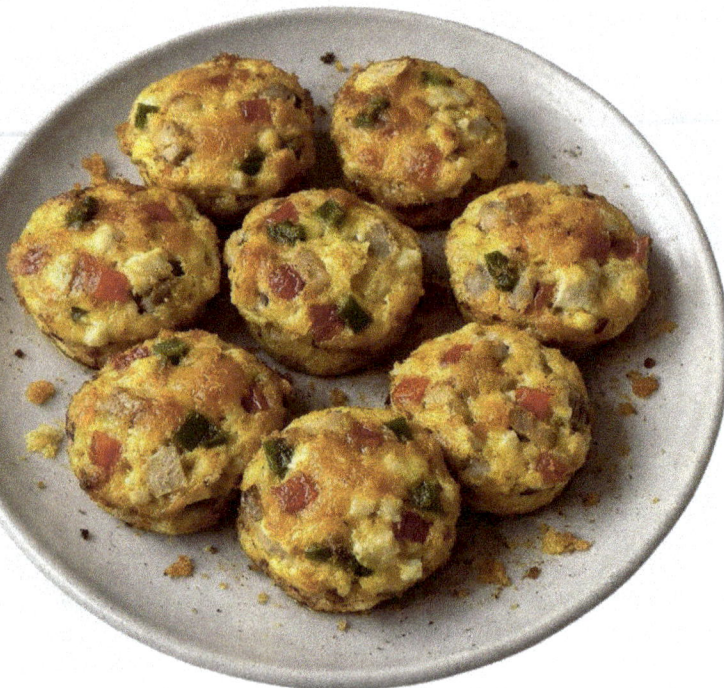

Servings 4

Prep Time 8'

Cook time 18'

COST PER RECIPE $8

GL 1/ LOW

NUTRITION (2 egg bites per serving)
Calories: 246 kcal | Protein: 21 g | Fat: 8 g | Carbohydrates: 6 g | Fiber: 1 g | Sodium: 228 mg

Creativity TWIST: Swap cheddar for mozzarella and bell peppers for spinach to make a "Florentine" version while keeping protein high and sodium low.

About this Recipe
Farmhouse-inspired warm egg bites deliver savory cheesy comfort, high-quality protein, lasting fullness, and balanced blood sugar support with each bite.

INGREDIENTS

- **8 large eggs**
- **1 cup low-fat cottage cheese**
- **1 cup reduced-fat shredded cheddar**
- **1 cup diced bell peppers (fresh or frozen)**
- **½ cup diced cooked turkey or chicken breast**
- **Optional seasonings: black pepper, garlic powder, onion powder**

DIRECTIONS

1. Preheat oven to 350°F (177°C) and spray a 12-cup muffin tin with cooking spray.
2. In a blender, puree eggs + cottage cheese until smooth.
3. Stir in cheddar, bell peppers, and diced turkey/chicken.
4. Pour mixture evenly into 8 muffin cups (leave 4 empty or fill with water for even baking).
5. Bake 17–18 minutes, or until set in the center.
6. Cool for 5 minutes before removing from the tin. Serve 2 egg bites per serving.

Farmhouse Vegie Breakfast Scramble

About this Recipe
Farmhouse vegetables and creamy eggs create a comforting scramble that feels nourishing, filling, and energizing.

INGREDIENTS

- 8 large eggs
- 1 cup low-fat, low-sodium cottage cheese
- 2 cups diced bell peppers & onions (fresh or frozen)
- 2 cups fresh spinach (or frozen, thawed and drained)
- 1 cup reduced-fat, low-sodium shredded cheddar

Optional seasonings: black pepper, garlic powder, onion powder, paprika

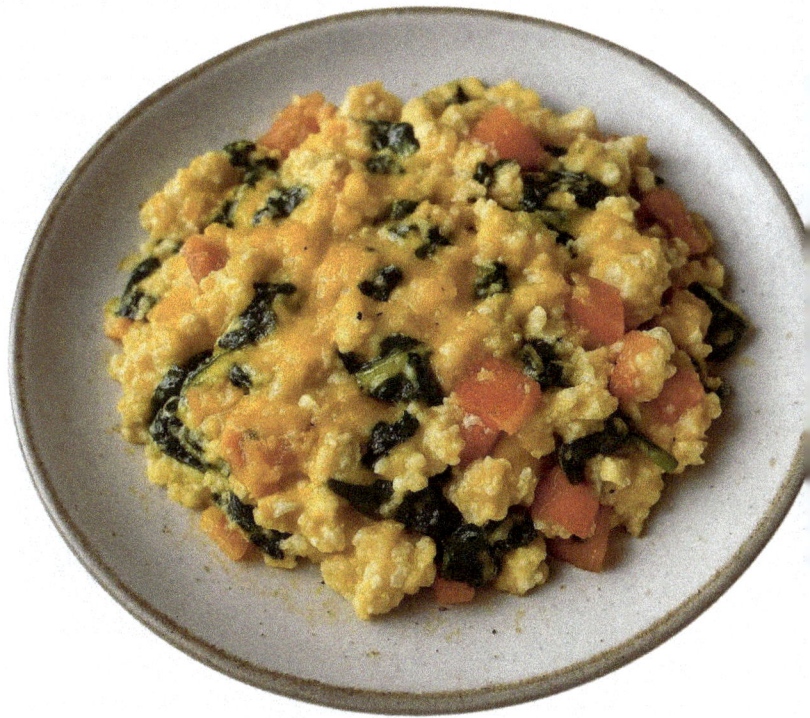

Servings **4**   Prep Time **7'**   Cook time **10'**

GL **1/ LOW**   COST PER RECIPE **$8**

DIRECTIONS

1. Spray a large skillet with cooking spray and heat over medium.
2. Add bell peppers & onions and sauté 3 minutes.
3. Add spinach and cook 2 minutes until wilted.
4. Whisk eggs and cottage cheese together in a bowl, then pour into the skillet.
5. Scramble gently until eggs are cooked through.
6. Stir in the cheddar until it melts and blends.

NUTRITION (1¼ cups per serving)
Calories: 312 kcal | Protein: 32 g | Fat: 13 g | Carbohydrates: 20 g | Fiber: 4 g | Sodium: 258 mg

Creativity TWIST: Swap cheddar for mozzarella and add mushrooms for an "omelet-style" version, or wrap the scramble in a whole-wheat tortilla to convert it into a 5-ingredient breakfast burrito.

Cheesy Black Bean Breakfast Quesadillas

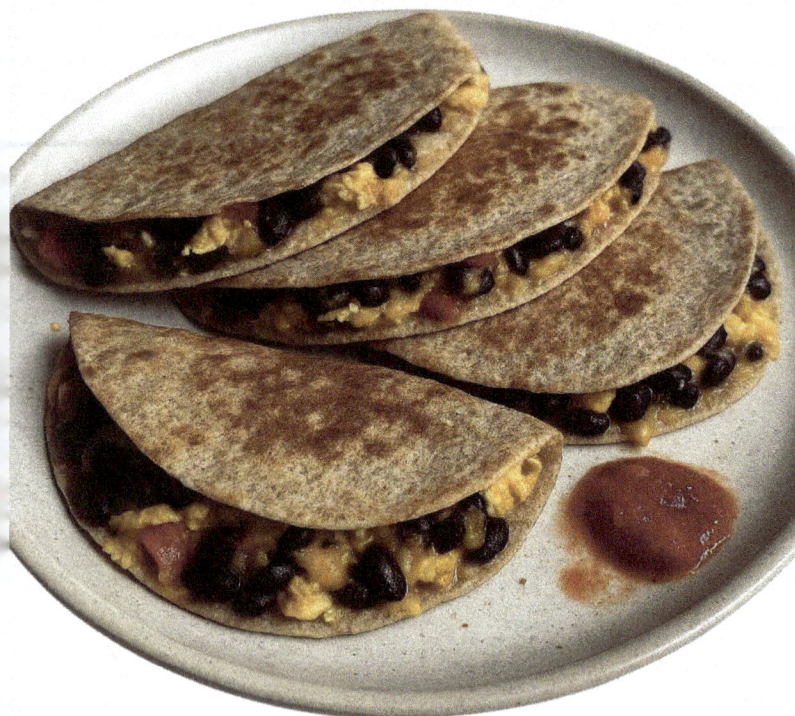

About this Recipe
Whole-grain tortillas and beans provide fiber-rich complex carbs that boost fullness and support weight loss and blood sugar control.

INGREDIENTS

- 4 whole-wheat tortillas
- 1 (15 oz) can low sodium black beans, rinsed and drained
- 4 large eggs
- 1 cup reduced-fat shredded cheddar
- 1 cup diced bell peppers (fresh or frozen)
- Optional seasonings: black pepper, onion powder, garlic powder, salsa (1 tbsp for flavor, ok)

Servings **4** Prep Time **8'** Cook time **8'**

COST PER RECIPE **$7** GL **12/ MID**

DIRECTIONS

1. Spray a skillet with cooking spray and heat over medium.
2. Add diced bell peppers and sauté 2–3 minutes.
3. Add eggs and scramble until fully cooked.
4. Stir in black beans and cheddar until warm and melted.
5. Divide the mixture evenly among 4 tortillas, fold in half, and return to the skillet.
6. Cook 2 minutes per side until lightly crisp.
7. Serve warm.

NUTRITION (1 quesadilla per serving)
Calories: 392 kcal | Protein: 28 g | Fat: 7 g | Carbohydrates: 42 g | Fiber: 10 g | Sodium: 284 mg

Creativity TWIST: Swap bell peppers for spinach to make a mild "Florentine" version, or add ¼ cup corn to the filling for texture without increasing sodium..

Crispy Turkey Bacon–Egg Quesadilla Melt

About this Recipe

Golden, crispy tortillas wrap smoky turkey bacon and eggs for a craveable, hearty bite that keeps you full.

INGREDIENTS

- 4 whole-wheat tortillas
- 6 large eggs
- 6 slices low-sodium turkey bacon (cooked and chopped)
- 1 cup reduced-fat shredded cheddar
- 4 tbsp salsa (1 tbsp per quesadilla)

Optional: black pepper, onion powder, garlic powder

DIRECTIONS

1. Spray a skillet with cooking spray and heat over medium.
2. Scramble eggs until fully cooked; season with optional black pepper.
3. Add chopped turkey bacon and cheddar to the skillet; heat until cheese begins to melt.
4. Divide filling evenly across 4 tortillas and fold in half.
5. Return the folded quesadillas to the skillet and cook for 2 minutes per side, until lightly crisp.
6. Serve warm with 1 tbsp salsa on top or inside each quesadilla.

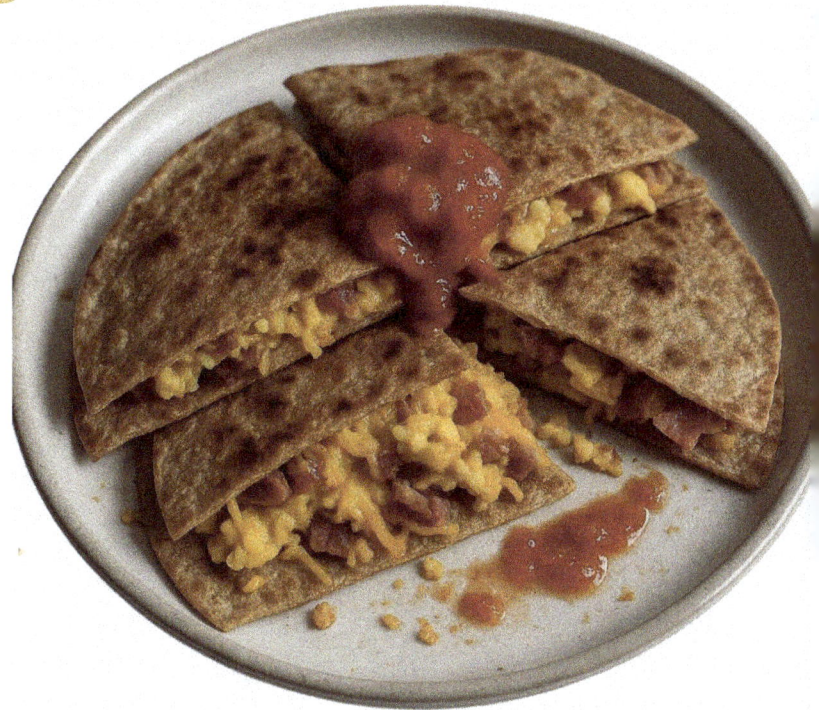

Servings	Prep Time	Cook time
4	8'	8'

GL	COST PER RECIPE
13/ MID	$9

NUTRITION (1 quesadilla per serving)

Calories: 398 kcal | Protein: 34 g | Fat: 8 g | Carbohydrates: 37 g | Fiber: 6 g | Sodium: 296 mg

Creativity TWIST: Swap salsa for diced tomatoes + green onions for lower sodium, or replace cheddar with pepper jack for a spicier version without adding salt.

Creamy Berry Nut Crunch Yogurt Parfait

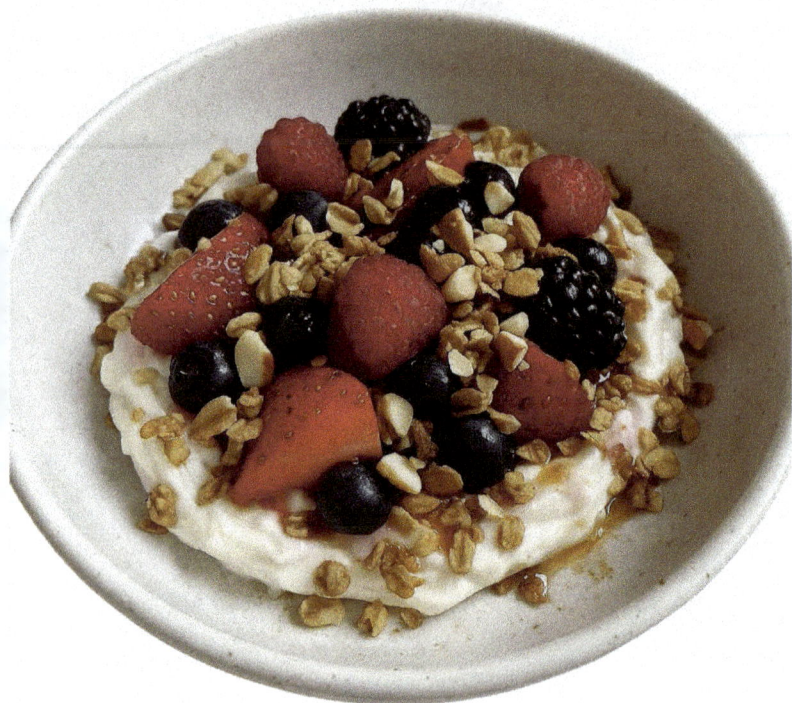

About this Recipe

Creamy yogurt, sweet berries, and crunchy nuts create a refreshing, satisfying parfait that energizes and keeps you full.

INGREDIENTS

- 3 cups non-fat Greek yogurt
- • 2 cups mixed berries (fresh or frozen)
- • ½ cup granola (whole-grain, low sugar preferred)
- • 2 tbsp sugar-free maple syrup
- • ¼ cup chopped almonds
- Optional: vanilla extract, cinnamon

Servings | Prep Time | Cook time
4 | 7' | 0'

COST PER RECIPE: $10

GL: 16/ MID

DIRECTIONS

1. Add ¾ cup Greek yogurt to 4 jars or bowls.
2. Top each with ½ cup berries.
3. Sprinkle 2 tbsp granola and 1 tbsp almonds over each parfait.
4. Drizzle ½ tbsp sugar-free syrup over each.
5. Serve immediately or refrigerate for up to 3 days (add granola just before serving if you want it to stay crunchy).

NUTRITION (1 cup per serving)
Calories: 312 kcal | Protein: 29 g | Fat: 4 g | Carbohydrates: 36 g | Fiber: 5 g | Sodium: 168 mg

Creativity TWIST: Swap berries for peaches and pineapple for a tropical version, or add 1 tbsp chia seeds for extra fiber and omega-3s without adding sodium.

Hearty Fruit & Fiber Muffins

About this Recipe
Soft, lightly sweet muffins burst with fruity flavor and feel hearty, comforting, and naturally satisfying.

INGREDIENTS

2 cups old-fashioned oats, ground into flour
• **2 cups unsweetened applesauce**
• **1 cup non-fat Greek yogurt**
• **1 cup mixed berries (fresh or frozen)**
• **⅓ cup chia seeds**

DIRECTIONS

1. Preheat oven to 350°F (177°C) and spray a 12-cup muffin tin with cooking spray.
2. Blend oats in a blender or food processor to create oat flour.
3. In a large bowl, combine oat flour, applesauce, Greek yogurt, and chia seeds.
4. Fold in berries gently.
5. Divide batter evenly into 6 muffin cups.
6. Bake 18–20 minutes, or until set and lightly golden.
7. Cool for 5 minutes, then serve 1 muffin per serving; refrigerate up to 5 days.

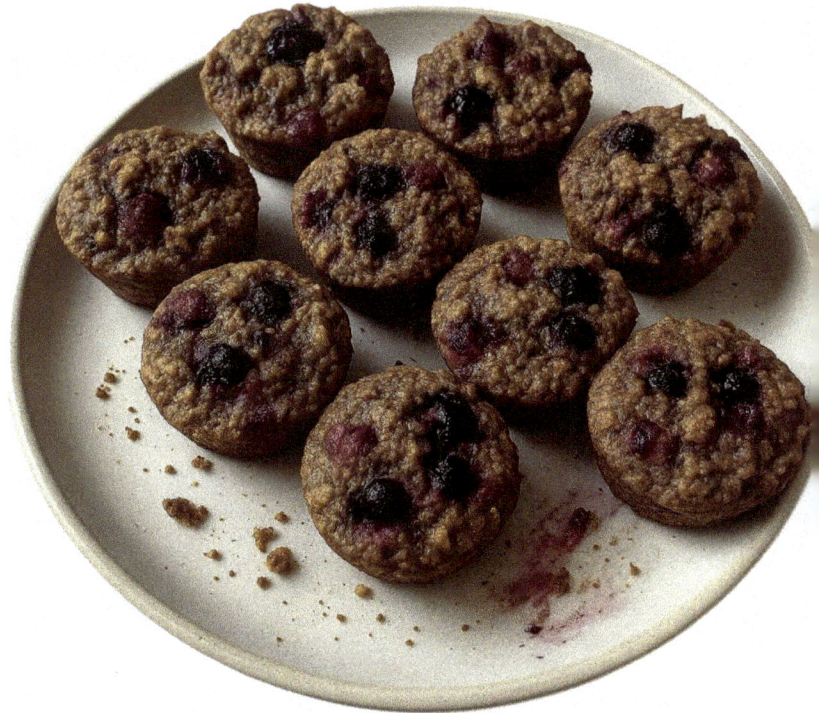

Servings: 6
Prep Time: 10'
Cook time: 20'
GL: 14/ MID
COST PER RECIPE: $10

NUTRITION 6 muffins (1 per serving)
Calories: 232 kcal | Protein: 9 g | Fat: 5 g | Carbohydrates: 36 g | Fiber: 8 g | Sodium: 16 mg

Creativity TWIST: Swap berries for peaches & cinnamon for a peach cobbler flavor, or use pumpkin puree instead of applesauce + cinnamon to turn this into a fall muffin without changing sodium.

Homestyle Oat Breakfast Bars

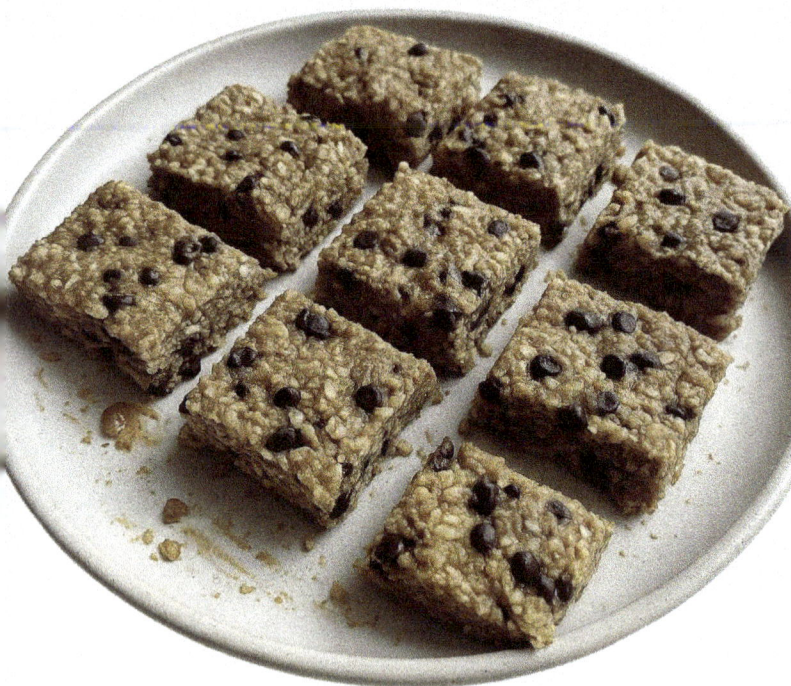

About this Recipe
Homestyle Oat Breakfast bars taste chewy, lightly sweet, and chocolatey with a cozy peanut-butter flavor that feels comforting.

INGREDIENTS

- 3 cups old-fashioned oats
- 1 cup powdered peanut butter (PB2 or similar)
- 1 cup non-fat Greek yogurt
- ½ cup sugar-free maple syrup
- ½ cup mini sugar-free chocolate chips
- Optional: cinnamon, vanilla extract

Servings: **8**   Prep Time: **10'**   Cook time: **0'**

COST PER RECIPE: **$9**   GL: **18/ MID**

DIRECTIONS

1. Line an 8×8 dish with parchment paper.
2. Add oats, powdered peanut butter, Greek yogurt, and sugar-free maple syrup to a bowl; mix well.
3. Fold the chocolate chips.
4. Press the mixture firmly into the baking dish.
5. Refrigerate 1–2 hours, then slice into 8 equal bars.
6. Serve.

NUTRITION (1 bar each)
Calories: 312 kcal | Protein: 18 g | Fat: 7 g | Carbohydrates: 39 g | Fiber: 6 g | Sodium: 164 mg

Creativity TWIST: Swap chocolate chips for blueberries for a fruity version, or add 1 scoop vanilla protein powder for even more protein without raising sodium.

Avocado Egg Protein Power Bowl

About this Recipe
Creamy avocado, fluffy quinoa, and eggs create a fresh, savory bowl that feels filling and energizing.

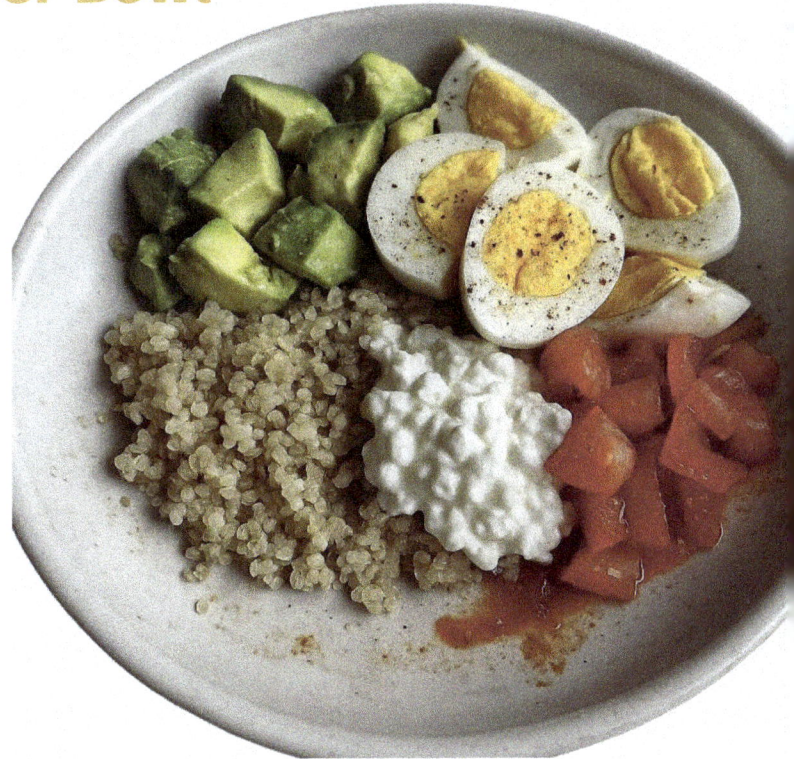

INGREDIENTS

- 6 large eggs
- 2 medium avocados, diced
- 2 cups cooked quinoa (plain)
- 1 cup non-fat cottage cheese
- 1 cup diced tomatoes

Optional seasonings: black pepper, garlic powder, onion powder, paprika, salsa (1 tbsp for flavor)

DIRECTIONS

1. Add quinoa to 4 bowls (½ cup each).
2. Hard-boil or soft-boil eggs (8 minutes for firm yolk).
3. Slice eggs and divide evenly among bowls.
4. Top each bowl with ½ avocado, ¼ cup cottage cheese, and ¼ cup tomatoes.
5. Sprinkle optional black pepper or paprika before serving.

Servings
4

Prep Time
10'

Cook time
8'

COST PER RECIPE
$9

GL
2/ LOW

NUTRITION (2 cups per serving)
Calories: 361 kcal | Protein: 22 g | Fat: 17 g | Carbohydrates: 29 g | Fiber: 6 g | Sodium: 133 mg

Creativity TWIST: Swap quinoa for brown rice for a milder flavor, or add 2 tbsp of black beans per serving to boost fiber while keeping sodium in check.

Quick Skillet Chicken Fajitas

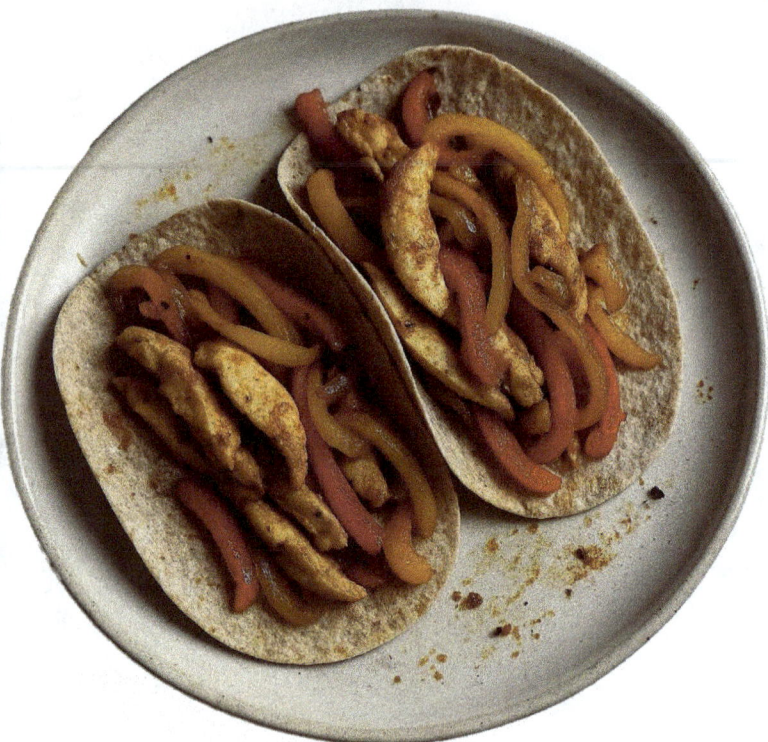

About this Recipe
Sizzling chicken mingles with peppers, smoky spice wrapped warmly in tortillas, bursting with juicy comfort.

INGREDIENTS

- 1½ lbs. chicken breast, sliced thin
- 2 tsp olive oil
- 4 cups sliced bell peppers & onions
- 2 tsp no-salt homemade fajita seasoning
- 8 small whole-wheat tortillas (2 per serving)

Servings **4** Prep Time **12'** Cook time **10'**

COST PER RECIPE **$10** GL **13/ MID**

DIRECTIONS

1. Heat olive oil in a skillet over medium-high heat.
2. Add the chicken; cook for 6–7 minutes, until browned.
3. Add peppers/onions; cook 6–7 minutes.
4. Stir in fajita seasoning; toss to coat.
5. Serve inside a warm tortilla.

NUTRITION (1 FAJITA)
Calories: 502 | Protein: 59 g | Fat: 12g | Carbohydrates: 38 g | Fiber: 7 g | Sodium: 426 mg

Creativity TWIST: Add lime juice and cilantro for flavor without increasing sodium; swap tortillas for lettuce cups for a low-carb version.

Recommended Side Dishes:
1. Fresh Green Salad p. 65
2. Brown Rice Pilaf p. 58

Tasty Teriyaki Turkey Meatballs

About this Recipe
Juicy turkey meatballs glazed with savory-sweet teriyaki deliver bold flavor, satisfying protein, and comforting warmth.

INGREDIENTS

- 2 lbs. lean ground turkey
- ½ cup rolled oats
- 2 eggs
- 1 tsp garlic powder
- 4 tbsp low-sodium teriyaki sauce (after cooking)

DIRECTIONS

1. Preheat oven to 400°F (200°C).
2. Mix turkey, oats, eggs, and garlic; roll into 32 meatballs.
3. Bake 18–20 minutes until browned.
4. Brush lightly with teriyaki sauce while hot.

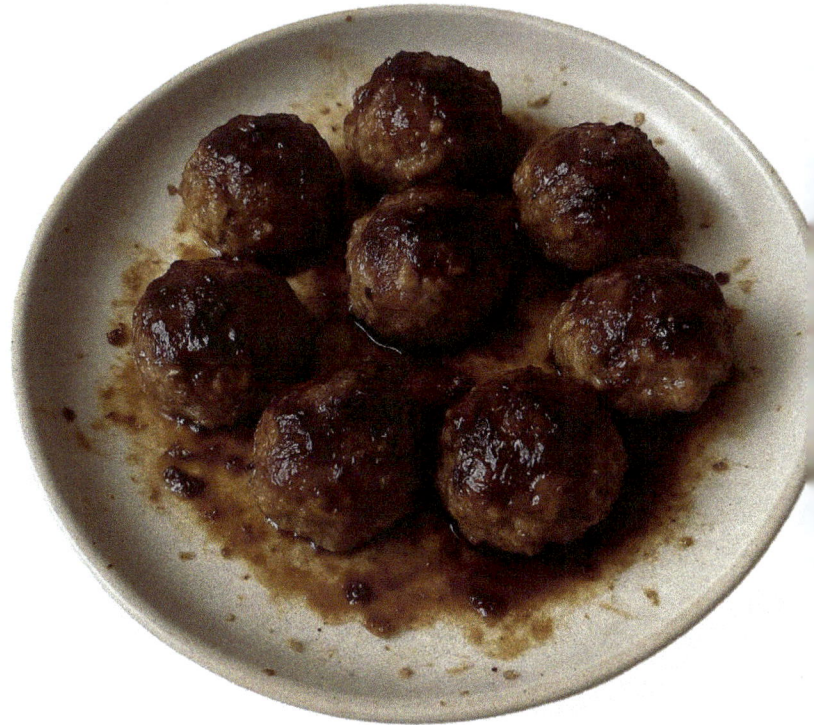

Servings **4** Prep Time **12'** Cook time **18'**

GL **11/ MID** COST PER RECIPE **$9**

NUTRITION PER 8 MEATBALLS
Calories: 421 | Protein: 41 g | Fat: 20 g | Carbohydrates: 9 g | Fiber: 1 g | Sodium: 513 mg

Recommended Side Dishes:
1. Brown rice pilaf p. 58   2. Roasted Carrots p. 68
3. Garlic Sautéed Mushroomsp. 66

Creativity TWIST: Add ginger or sesame seeds to deepen flavor without adding sodium.

Cozy Chicken Noodle Casserole

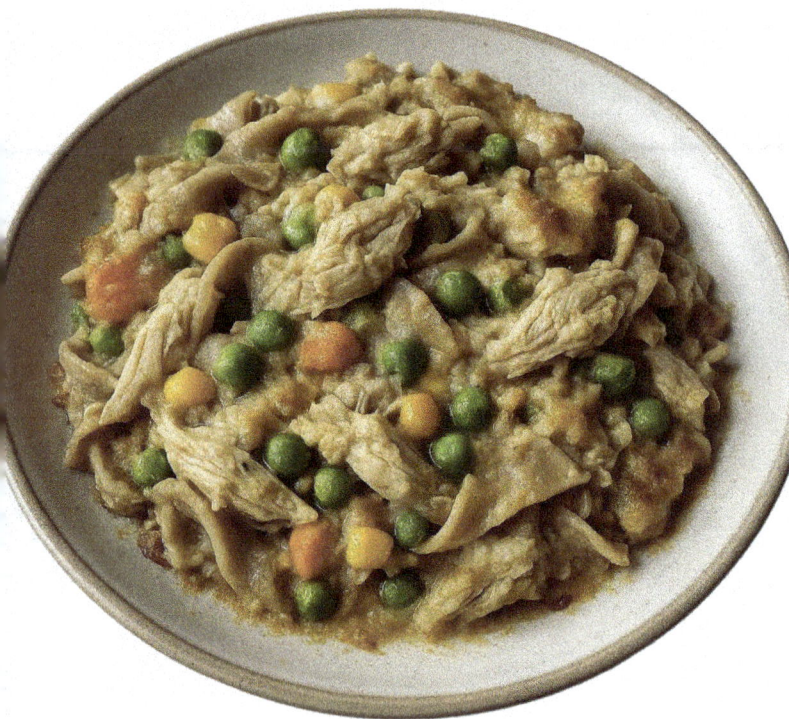

About this Recipe

Sizzling chicken mingles with peppers, smoky spice wrapped warmly in tortillas, bursting with juicy comfort.

INGREDIENTS

- 4 cups cooked whole-wheat egg noodles
- 4 cups cooked, shredded chicken breast
- 3 cups mixed vegetables
- 1 batch Homemade Cream of Chicken Soup (3 cups total)
- 1 tsp garlic powder

Servings: **4** Prep Time: **15'** Cook time: **28'**

COST PER RECIPE: **$9** GL: **11/ MID**

NUTRITION (1 cup per serving)
Calories: 372 kcal | Protein: 31 g | Fat: 6 g | Carbohydrates: 42 g | Fiber: 4 g | Sodium: 298 mg

DIRECTIONS

1. Preheat oven to 375°F (190°C).
2. In a large bowl, combine cooked noodles, shredded chicken, mixed vegetables, garlic powder, and the full batch of Homemade Cream of Chicken Soup.
3. Spread mixture evenly into a casserole dish.
4. Bake 28–32 minutes, or until hot and lightly golden on top.
5. Scoop 1 cup per serving. Let it rest for 5 minutes before serving.

Creativity TWIST: Top casserole with ¼ cup whole-wheat breadcrumbs for a crispy finish (+4 g carbs per serving). For extra creaminess, stir in ¼ cup non-fat Greek yogurt after baking, not before, to prevent separation.

Recommended Side Dishes:
1. Fresh Green Salad p. 65

Zesty Lemon Chicken

About this Recipe
Classic comfort flavors come together in a warm, creamy bake that feels nourishing, satisfying, and cozy.

INGREDIENTS

- 1½ lbs. boneless, skinless chicken breasts (thinly sliced)
- 2 tsp olive oil
- 4 tbsp lemon juice (fresh preferred)
- 2 tsp garlic powder
- 1 tsp dried Italian seasoning (optional))

DIRECTIONS

1. Heat olive oil in a large skillet over medium-high heat.
2. Season chicken with garlic and Italian seasoning.
3. Cook 5–6 minutes per side, until lightly browned and internal temperature reaches 165°F.
4. Add lemon juice in the final minute of cooking and spoon sauce over chicken before serving.

Servings 4 | Prep Time 10' | Cook time 15'

GL 5/ LOW | COST PER RECIPE $6

NUTRITION 4 OZ per serving
Calories: 258 | Protein: 35 g | Fat: 8 g | Carbohydrates: 4 g | Fiber: 0 g | Sodium: 212 mg

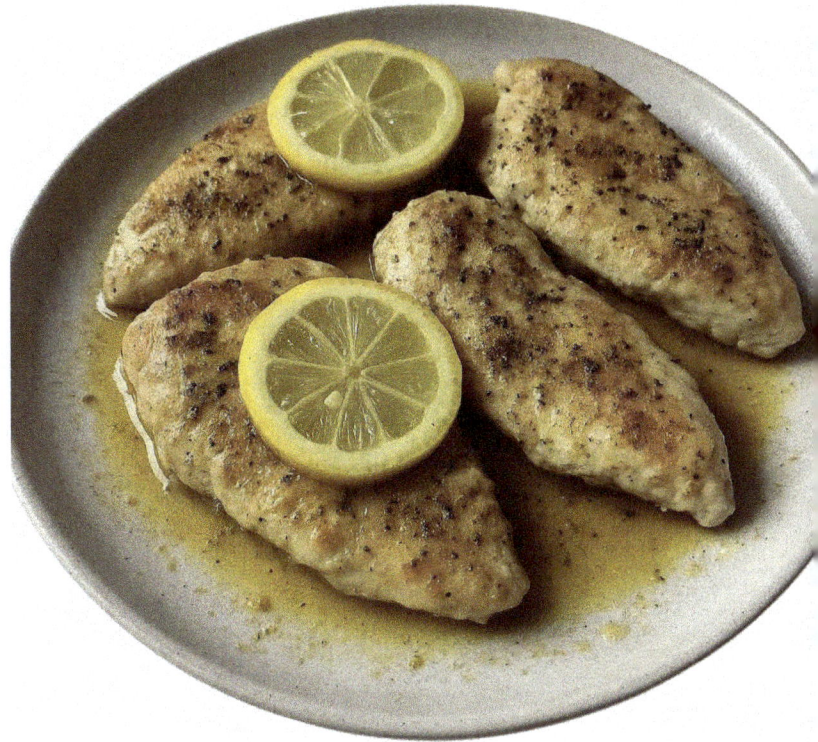

Recommended Side Dishes:
1. Parmesan Risotto p. 57 2. Creamy Cheesy Broccoli Couscous p. 70 3. Roasted Green Beans with Tomatoes p. 62 4. Oven Roasted Broccoli with Parmesan p. 60

Creativity TWIST: Finish with an extra squeeze of fresh lemon and a sprinkle of chopped parsley for brightness.
Add a pinch of red chili flakes in the final minute for a subtle, zesty kick.

Quick and Crispy Salmon Patties

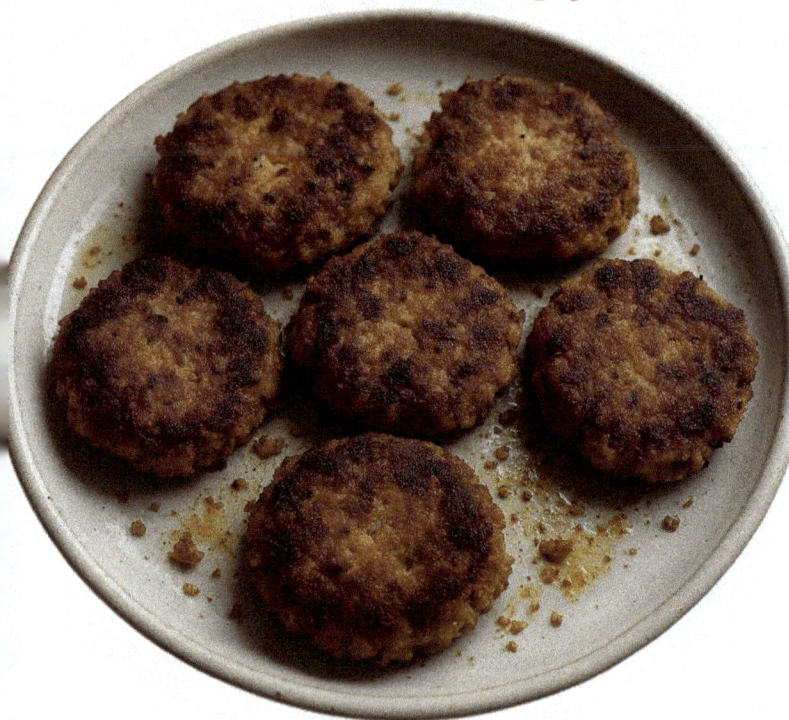

About this Recipe
Golden, crispy salmon patties offer savory flavor with satisfying protein and a comforting, home-style bite.

INGREDIENTS

- 2 cans (14.75 oz each) salmon, drained & flaked
- 2 eggs
- 1 cup whole-wheat breadcrumbs
- 1 tsp garlic powder
- 2 tsp olive oil (for pan-frying)

DIRECTIONS

1. In a bowl, combine salmon, eggs, breadcrumbs, and garlic powder; mix well.
2. Shape mixture into 8 patties.
3. Heat olive oil in a skillet over medium heat.
4. Cook patties 3–4 minutes per side, until golden brown.
5. Serve warm.

Servings 4 | Prep Time 10' | Cook time 12'

COST PER RECIPE $9 | GL 8/ LOW

NUTRITION (2 PATTIES PER SERVING)
Calories: 362 | Protein: 30 g | Fat: 11 g | Carbohydrates: 22 g | Fiber: 2 g | Sodium: 352 mg

Creativity TWIST: Add lemon zest and fresh dill to the mixture for a bright coastal flavor without increasing sodium; swap breadcrumbs for rolled oats for extra fiber; or turn the patties into "salmon sliders" by serving on whole-grain mini buns with a thin spread of Greek yogurt-dill sauce.

Recommended Side Dishes:
1. Whole Grain Orzo with Spinach & Parmesan p. 69
2. Roasted Zucchini & Summer Squash p. 62

Creamy Tuna Noodle Casserole

About this Recipe
Creamy, comforting tuna noodles deliver classic flavor with satisfying protein and a cozy, nostalgic bite.

INGREDIENTS

- 4 cups cooked whole-wheat egg noodles
- 2 cans (5 oz each) tuna in water, drained
- 3 cups mixed vegetables
- 1 batch Homemade Cream of Chicken Soup (3 cups total)
- 1 tsp Mrs. Dash Table Blend (or homemade salt-free seasoning)

DIRECTIONS

1. Preheat oven to 375°F (190°C).
2. In a large bowl, combine cooked noodles, tuna, mixed vegetables, and the full batch of Homemade Cream of Chicken Soup.
3. Add Mrs. Dash Table Blend and mix until well combined.
4. Spread mixture evenly into a casserole dish.
5. Bake 28–32 minutes, or until hot and lightly golden.
6. Serve 1 cup per portion and allow it to rest for 5 minutes before serving.

Recommended Side Dishes:
1. Fresh Green Salad p. 65

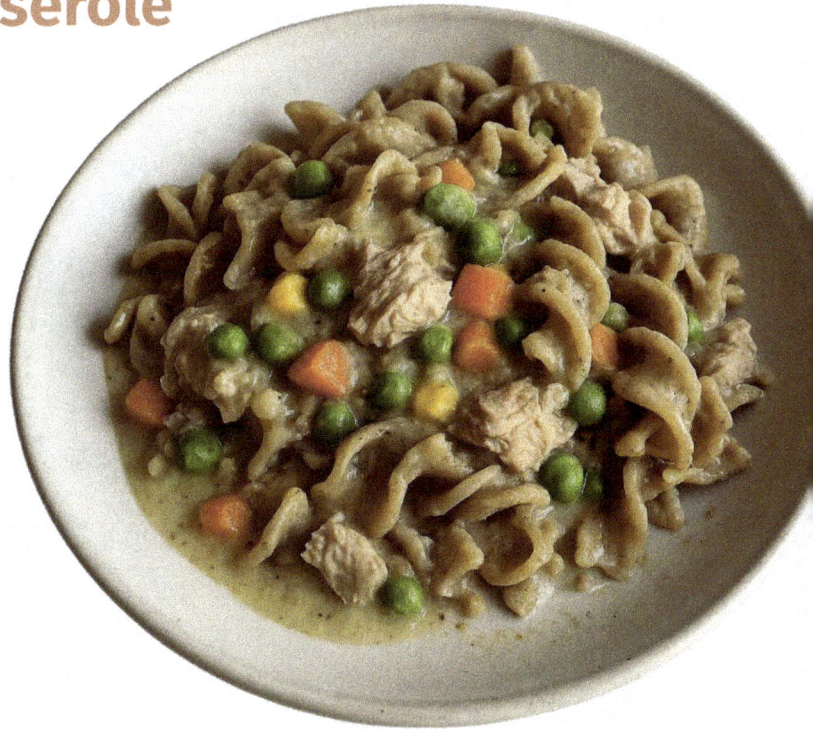

Servings	Prep Time	Cook time
4	15'	28'

GL	COST PER RECIPE
11/ MID	$8

NUTRITION (2 cups per serving)
Calories: 368 kcal | Protein: 30 g | Fat: 6 g | Carbohydrates: 40 g | Fiber: 6 g | Sodium: 180 mg

Creativity TWIST: Sprinkle ¼ cup whole-wheat breadcrumbs on top before baking for a crisp finish (+4 g carbs per serving) or add a squeeze of lemon after baking to brighten flavor without increasing sodium.

Homemade Cream of Chicken Soup

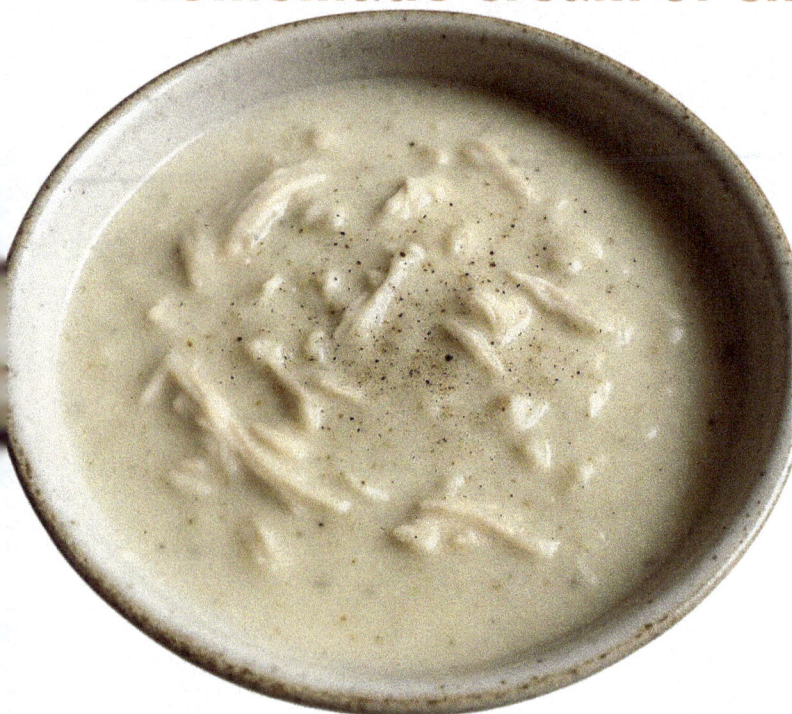

About this Recipe
A light, homemade cream soup made with simple, wholesome ingredients and great comfort flavor.

INGREDIENTS

- 2 cups of low-sodium chicken broth
- 1 cup non-fat milk (or 2% milk for creamier texture)
- ½ cup shredded cooked chicken breast
- ¼ cup all-purpose flour
- 1 tsp garlic powder
- 1 tsp onion powder
- ¼ tsp black pepper

Servings
8

Prep Time
8'

Cook time
10'

COST PER RECIPE
$2

GL
8/ LOW

DIRECTIONS

1. In a saucepan, whisk chicken broth and milk together over medium heat.
2. Add the flour, garlic powder, onion powder, and black pepper, whisking until smooth.
3. Continue heating, stirring frequently, until mixture thickens (about 8–10 minutes).
4. Stir in cooked, shredded chicken.
5. Remove from heat and serve warm (¾ cup per serving) or use in casseroles.

NUTRITION (¾ CUP EACH)
Calories: 156 kcal | Protein: 12 g | Fat: 5 g | Carbohydrates: 14 g | Fiber: 0 g | Sodium: 165 mg

Creativity TWIST: For extra depth, add a pinch of dried thyme or poultry seasoning while the soup thickens. For a silkier texture, whisk in 1–2 tablespoons non-fat Greek yogurt after removing from heat.

Recommended Side Dishes:
1. Whole Grain Orzo with Spinach & Parmesan p. 69
2. Roasted Zucchini p. 79 & Summer Squashp. 67

Homestyle Beef and Noodles

About this Recipe
Rich, savory beef and tender noodles create a hearty, comforting dish that feels filling and satisfying.

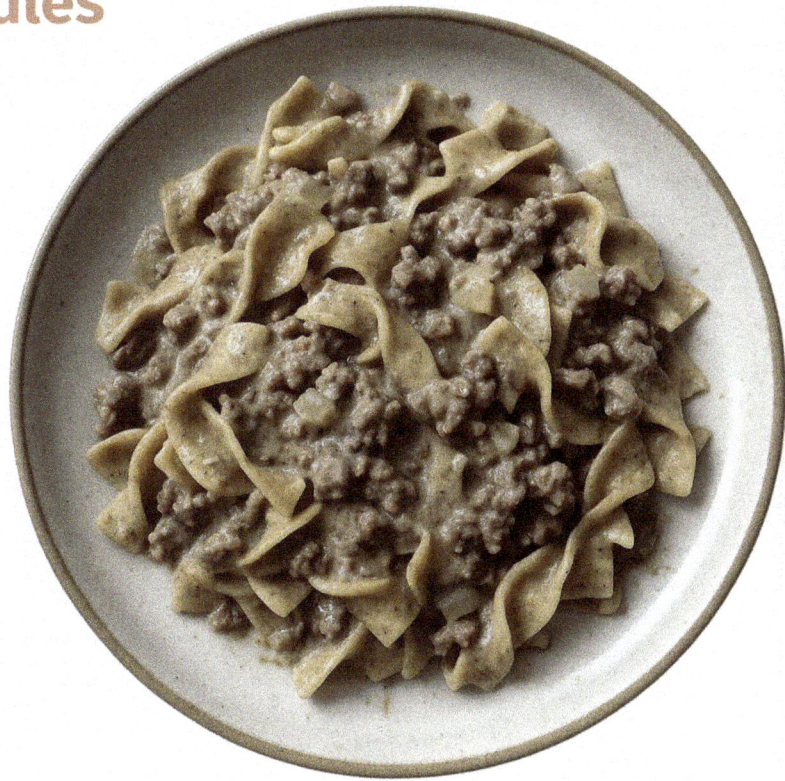

INGREDIENTS

- 1 lb. ground beef (85% lean), cooked, drained & rinsed to reduce fat
- 4 cups cooked whole-wheat egg noodles
- 1 batch Homemade Cream of Mushroom Soup (3 cups total)
- 1 tbsp Worcestershire sauce (reduced sodium if available)
- ½ tsp black pepper
- (Optional) ½ cup chopped onion

DIRECTIONS

1. Brown ground beef in a skillet over medium heat for 7–8 minutes.
2. Drain well and rinse under hot water to reduce fat, then return to the skillet.
3. (If using onions) Add chopped onion and cook 3–4 minutes until softened.
4. Add the full batch of Homemade Cream of Mushroom Soup and stir well.
5. Mix in Worcestershire sauce and black pepper.
6. Add cooked noodles and fold gently until creamy and evenly combined.
7. Serve warm (1 cup per serving) and allow it to rest 5 minutes before eating.

Recommended Side Dishes:

1. Roasted Broccoli with Parmesan p. 60
2. Roasted Carrots p. 68

Servings	Prep Time	Cook time
4	15'	25'

GL	COST PER RECIPE
19/ MID	$10

NUTRITION (1 CUP PER SERVING)
Calories: 448 kcal | Protein: 36 g | Fat: 10 g | Carbohydrates: 46 g | Fiber: 4 g | Sodium: 336 mg

Creativity TWIST: Swap ground beef for shredded roast, add 1 cup frozen peas for color and fiber, and stir in ¼ cup Greek yogurt at the end for a creamy, high-protein finish without extra sodium.

Homemade Cream of Mushroom Soup

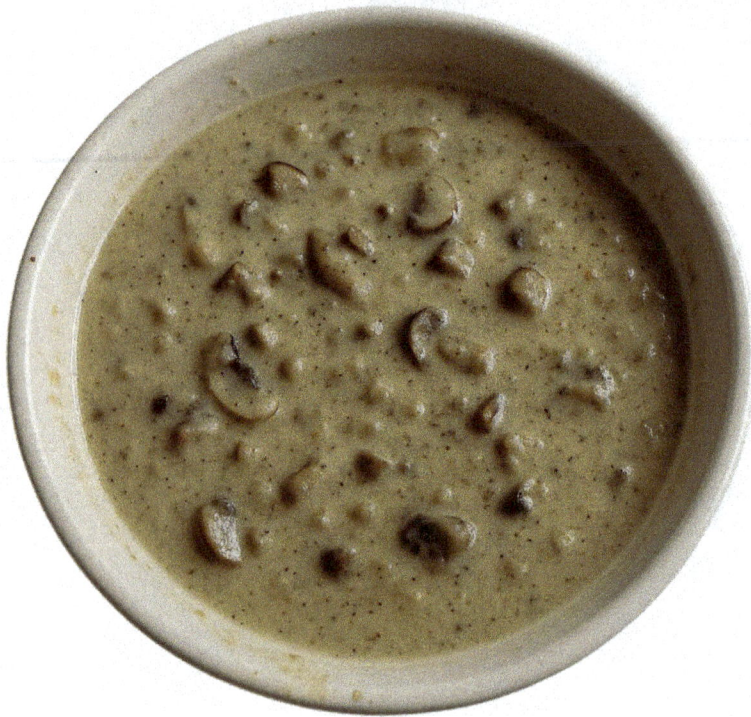

About this Recipe

A lighter, homemade cream of mushroom soup with rich, earthy flavor—perfect for casseroles, sauces, or cozy meals.

INGREDIENTS

- 2 cups low-sodium chicken broth (or vegetable broth for vegetarian version)
- 1 cup non-fat milk (or 2% milk for creamier texture)
- 1½ cups finely chopped mushrooms (button or baby belle)
- ¼ cup all-purpose flour
- 1 tsp Mrs. Dash Table Blend (or homemade salt-free seasoning)

DIRECTIONS

1. Add mushrooms to a non-stick skillet and cook on medium heat 4–5 minutes until softened (no oil needed).
2. In a saucepan, whisk broth and milk together over medium heat.
3. Slowly whisk in flour until smooth.
4. Add softened mushrooms and Mrs. Dash Table Blend.
5. Cook 8–10 minutes, stirring frequently, until soup thickens.
6. Serve warm (¾ cup per serving) or use as a casserole base.

Servings 4 | Prep Time 10' | Cook time 15'

COST PER RECIPE $5 | GL 5/ MID

NUTRITION (¾ CUP PER SERVING)
Calories: 152 kcal | Protein: 9 g | Fat: 4 g | Carbohydrates: 15 g | Fiber: 1 g | Sodium: 168 mg

Creativity TWIST: Add ¼ cup non-fat Greek yogurt for extra creaminess without raising sodium; or use a mix of baby Bella + shiitake mushrooms for a richer flavor while keeping carbs the same.

Wholesome Turkey Nourish Bowl

About this Recipe

Seasoned turkey, hearty grains, and colorful veggies come together in a balanced bowl that feels nourishing and satisfying.

INGREDIENTS

- 1 lb. lean ground turkey (93% lean)
- 2 tsp black pepper and garlic powder
- 2 cups of cooked brown rice
- 2 cups frozen peppers & onions
- 1 cup corn (fresh or frozen, thawed)
- 1 cup reduced-fat shredded cheddar cheese

DIRECTIONS

1. Heat the skillet over medium heat. Add ground turkey and cook 7–8 minutes, breaking it apart as it browns.
2. Drain excess liquid if needed. Season with black pepper and garlic pepper to taste.
3. In a second skillet, sauté frozen peppers and onions 4–5 minutes, until heated through.
4. Divide cooked brown rice into 4 bowls (½ cup each).
5. Top each with peppers/onions, corn, seasoned turkey, and cheddar cheese.
6. Serve warm.

Recommended Side Dishes:

1. Fresh Green Salad p. 65

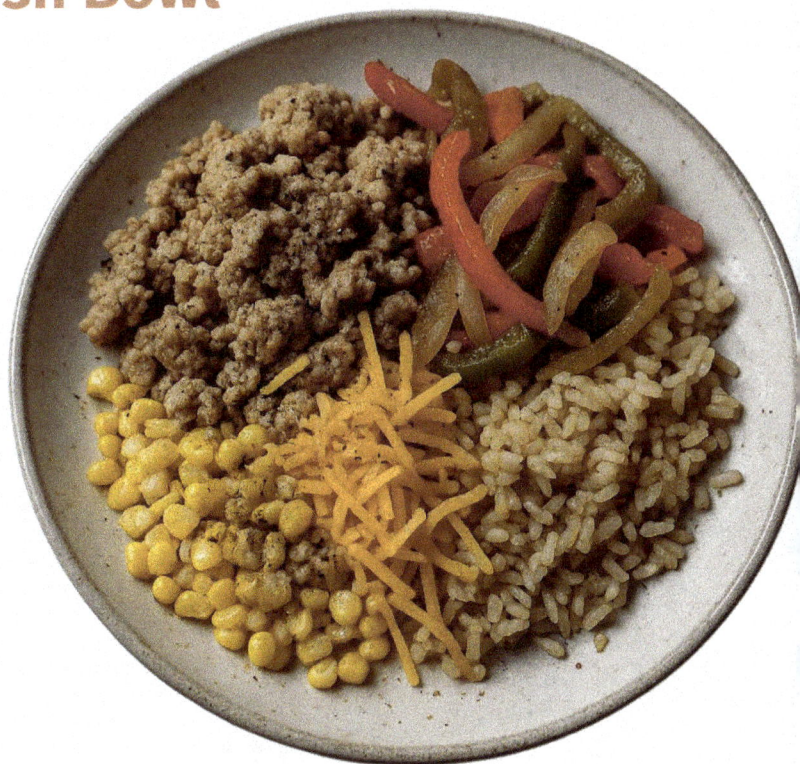

Servings	Prep Time	Cook time
4	12'	15'

GL	COST PER RECIPE
23/ HIGH	$10

NUTRITION (2 CUPS PER SERVING)
Calories: 466 kcal | Protein: 34 g | Fat: 15 g | Carbohydrates: 37 g | Fiber: 6 g | Sodium: 345 mg

Creativity TWIST: For an Italian version, replace cheddar with mozzarella and add chopped basil; for Mediterranean style, swap rice with farro and top with cucumber and tomato; for extra protein, add a dollop of non-fat Greek yogurt on top.

Zesty Lemon Pepper Tilapia

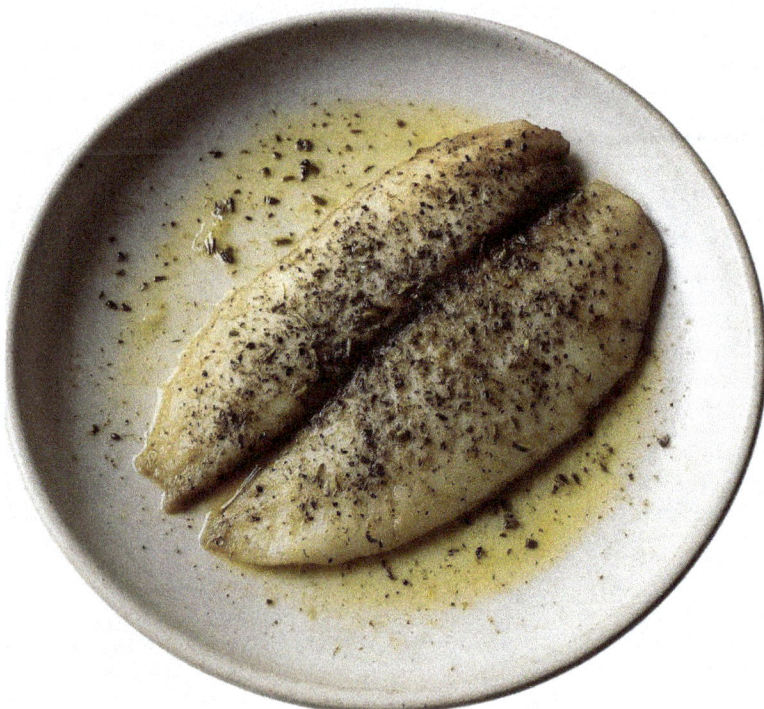

About this Recipe
Bright lemon and pepper enhance tender tilapia, creating a light, flavorful dish that feels fresh and satisfying.

INGREDIENTS

- 4 tilapia fillets (about 5–6 oz each)
- 2 tbsp lemon juice
- 1 tsp black pepper
- 1 tsp Italian seasoning (salt-free)
- 1 tsp minced garlic (optional)

Servings **4**   Prep Time **7'**   Cook time **14'**

COST PER RECIPE **$9**   GL **3/ LOW**

DIRECTIONS

1. Preheat oven to 400°F (204°C).
2. Place tilapia fillets on a parchment-lined baking sheet.
3. Drizzle lemon juice over the fish and rub gently with minced garlic if using.
4. Sprinkle with black pepper and Italian seasoning.
5. Bake 12–14 minutes, or until fish flakes easily with a fork.
6. Serve warm (1 fillet per serving)

NUTRITION (1 FILLET PER SERVING)
Calories: 186 kcal | Protein: 33 g | Fat: 4 g | Carbohydrates: 4 g | Fiber: 1 g | Sodium: 176 mg

Creativity TWIST: Sprinkle with 1 tbsp grated parmesan in the last 2 minutes of baking for a lightly browned topping, or serve over a bed of steamed broccoli or cauliflower rice to keep sodium and carbs low.

Recommended Side Dishes:
1. Roasted Asparagus with Lemon p. 61
2. Wild Rice Pilaf p. 59

Quick and Easy Creamy Garlic Pork Chops

About this Recipe
Tender pork chops simmered in creamy garlic sauce deliver rich comfort that feels hearty yet balanced.

INGREDIENTS

- 4 boneless pork chops (about 5–6 oz each, trimmed of fat)
- 1 batch Homemade Cream of Chicken Soup (3 cups total)
- 1 cup low-fat milk (to thin the sauce)
- 1 tbsp minced garlic (fresh or jarred)
- ½ tsp black pepper)

DIRECTIONS

1. Preheat oven to 375°F (190°C).
2. Spray a skillet with cooking spray. Sear pork chops 2–3 minutes per side until lightly golden.
3. In a bowl, whisk together Homemade Cream of Chicken Soup, milk, minced garlic, and black pepper.
4. Place pork chops in a baking dish and pour the creamy sauce over the top.
5. Cover with foil and bake for 20 minutes, or until pork reaches 145°F internal temperature.
6. Serve one pork chop with ⅓–½ cup of sauce per serving.

Recommended Side Dishes:
1. Garlic Mashed Potatoes p. 56
2. Roasted Broccoli with Parmesan p. 60

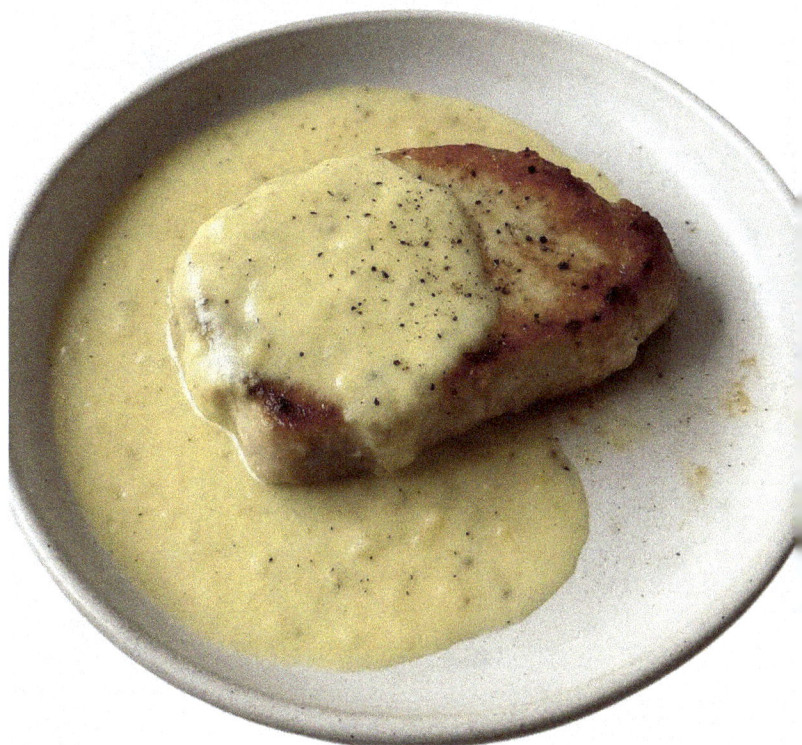

Servings 4 | Prep Time 12' | Cook time 20'

GL 4/ LOW | COST PER RECIPE $10

NUTRITION (1 CHOP PER SERVING)
Calories: 313 kcal | Protein: 37 g | Fat: 12 g | Carbohydrates: 8 g | Fiber: 1 g | Sodium: 189 mg

Creativity TWIST: Add ¼ cup non-fat Greek yogurt after baking for a silky, stroganoff-style finish.

Homestyle Garlic Mashed Potatoes with Skin

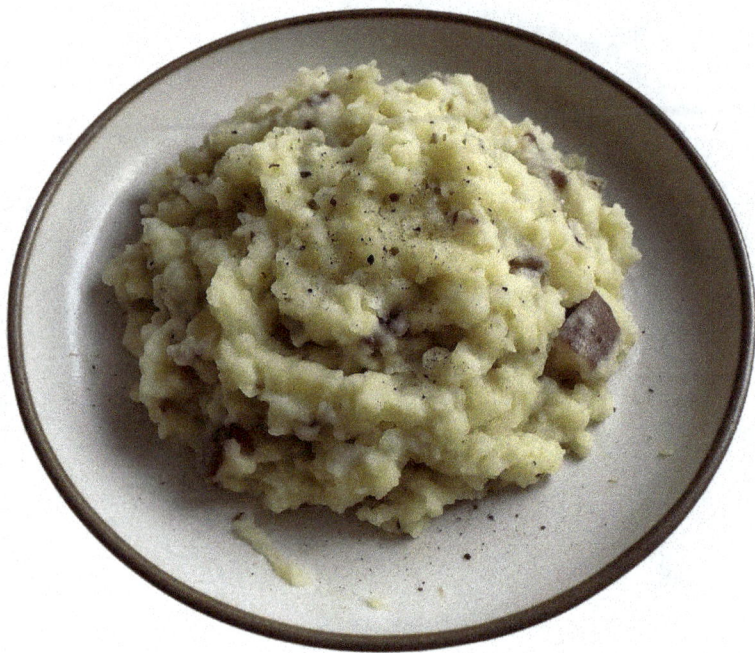

About this Recipe
Rustic potatoes mashed creamy, garlicky warmth, skins whispering earthiness, inviting slow, comforting bites at dinner.

INGREDIENTS

- **3 lbs. red potatoes (skins on, washed & diced)**
- • **¾ cup skim milk (or 2% if preferred)**
- • **¼ cup light sour cream**
- • **1 tbsp olive oil**
- • **1 tbsp minced garlic (fresh or jarred)**
- **Optional: black pepper, parsley, garlic powder**

Servings 6
Prep Time 10'
Cook time 20'

COST PER RECIPE $6
GL 18/ MID

NUTRITION (1 CUP PER SERVING)
Calories: 202 kcal | Pr otein: 5 g | Fat: 4 g | Carbohydrates: 40 g | Fiber: 4 g | Sodium: 39 mg

Creativity TWIST: For extra creaminess without extra fat, stir in ¼ cup plain Greek yogurt — it increases protein while keeping sodium low. Or sprinkle 2 tbsp shredded Parmesan on top right before serving (adds savory flavor without much fat).

DIRECTIONS

1. Add diced potatoes to a pot, cover with water, and bring them to a boil.
2. Reduce heat and simmer 18–20 minutes or until fork-tender.
3. Drain and return potatoes to the warm pot.
4. Add garlic, milk, sour cream, and olive oil.
5. Mash to desired consistency — smooth or slightly chunky with skins visible.
6. Season with optional black pepper and serve warm.
7. Serving size = 1 cup

Creamy Parmesan Risotto

About this Recipe

Slow-stirred rice and Parmesan create a luxuriously creamy risotto that feels comforting, rich, and satisfying.

INGREDIENTS

- 1 ½ cups arborio rice
- 5 cups low-sodium chicken broth (warmed)
- 1 cup skim milk
- ¾ cup grated Parmesan cheese (reduced-fat if available)
- 1 cup finely diced onion
- Optional: black pepper, garlic powder, parsley, olive oil spray

DIRECTIONS

1. Spray a large pot lightly with cooking spray and heat over medium.
2. Add diced onion and cook 3–4 minutes until softened.
3. Add arborio rice and stir 1 minute to lightly toast.
4. Add 1 cup warm broth, stirring constantly until absorbed.
5. Continue adding broth ½–1 cup at a time, stirring until absorbed before each addition.
6. When all broth is absorbed, and rice is creamy, stir in milk and Parmesan.
7. Season with optional black pepper and serve.
8. Serving size = 1 cup

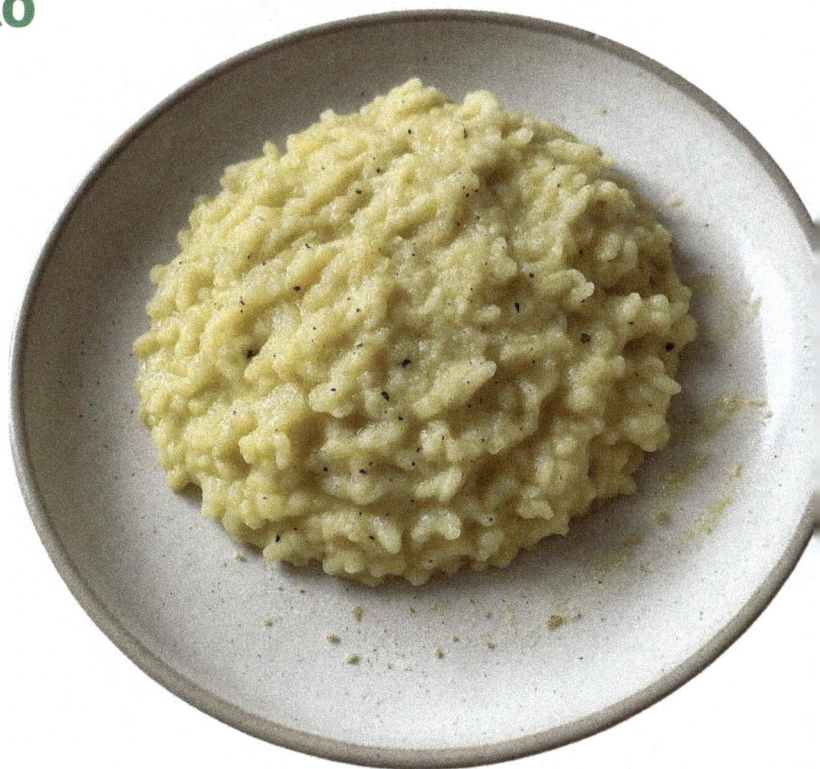

Servings **6** Prep Time **10'** Cook time **25'**

GL **22/ HIGH** COST PER RECIPE **$8**

NUTRITION (1 CUP EACH)
Calories: 298 kcal | Protein: 12 g | Fat: 6 g | Carbohydrates: 38 g | Fiber: 2 g | Sodium: 186 mg

Creativity TWIST: Add 1 cup of peas at the end for color and texture (adds 4 g carbs per serving). For a protein boost, stir in 1 cup diced cooked chicken or shrimp. For vegetarian risotto, use vegetable broth instead of chicken.

Savory Brown Rice Pilaf

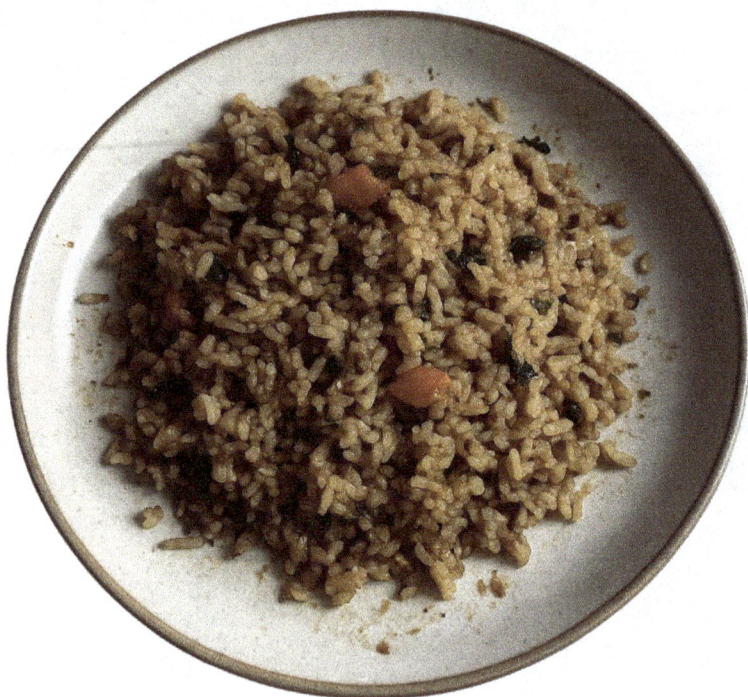

Servings	Prep Time	Cook time
6	8'	35'

COST PER RECIPE	GL
$5	22/ HIGH

NUTRITION (1 CUP PER SERVING)
Calories: 262 kcal | Protein: 6 g | Fat: 4 g | Carbohydrates: 38 g | Fiber: 4 g | Sodium: 128 mg

Creativity TWIST: Add 1 cup frozen peas in the last 5 minutes of cooking for extra color and fiber (+4 g carbs per serving). Add ¼ cup slivered almonds after cooking for crunch and healthy fats. For a Mediterranean flavor, stir in lemon zest + parsley before serving.

About this Recipe
Nutty brown rice with tender vegetables creates a savory, comforting pilaf that feels wholesome and satisfying.

INGREDIENTS

- 2 cups brown rice (dry, uncooked)
- 4 cups low-sodium chicken broth (or vegetable broth)
- 1 cup diced onion
- 1 cup diced carrots
- 1 tbsp olive oil
- Optional: garlic powder, black pepper, parsley, thyme

DIRECTIONS

1. Heat olive oil in a large pot over medium heat.
2. Add diced onion and diced carrots; sauté 4–5 minutes until softened.
3. Stir in brown rice and cook 1 minute to lightly toast.
4. Pour in low-sodium broth and bring to a boil.
5. Reduce heat to low, cover, and simmer 35 minutes or until rice is tender and broth is absorbed.
6. Fluff with a fork, season with optional black pepper or parsley, and serve.

Hearty Wild Rice Pilaf

About this Recipe
Earthy wild rice and mushrooms create a hearty, rustic pilaf that feels nourishing, cozy, and deeply satisfying.

INGREDIENTS

- 2 cups wild rice blend (dry, uncooked)
- • 4 cups low-sodium vegetable broth (or chicken broth)
- • 1 cup diced onion
- • 1 cup diced mushrooms
- • 1 tbsp olive oil
- Optional: black pepper, thyme, garlic powder, parsley

DIRECTIONS

1. Heat olive oil in a large pot over medium heat.
2. Add diced onion and mushrooms; sauté 5 minutes until softened.
3. Add wild rice and stir for 1 minute to lightly toast.
4. Pour in low-sodium broth and bring to a boil.
5. Reduce the heat to low, cover, and simmer for 45 minutes or until the liquid is absorbed and the rice is tender.
6. Fluff with a fork and season with optional pepper or thyme.
7. Serving size = 1 cup

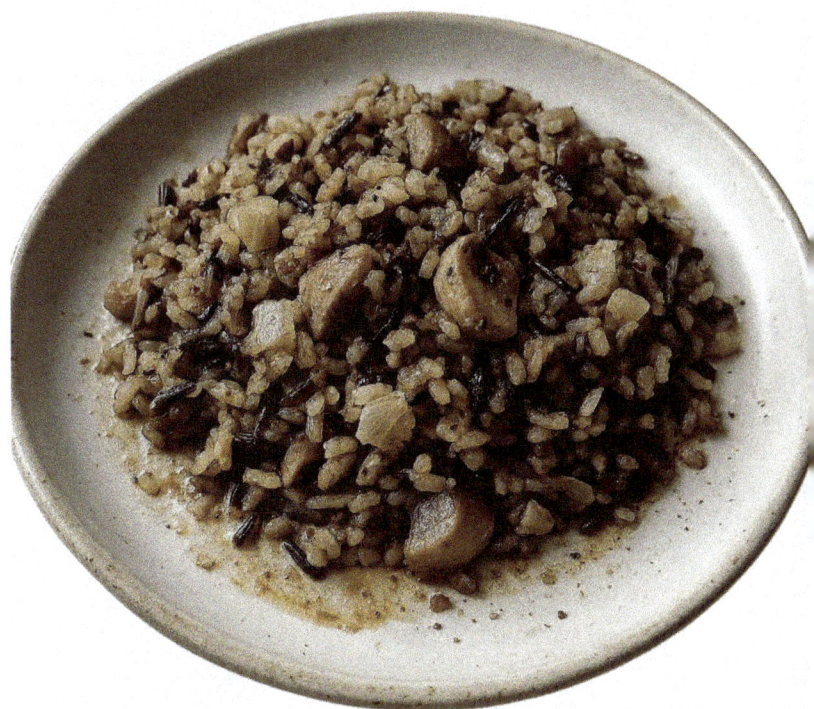

Servings 6 | Prep Time 8' | Cook time 45'

GL 16/ MID | COST PER RECIPE $8

NUTRITION (1 CUP EACH)
Calories: 268 kcal | Protein: 7 g | Fat: 4 g | Carbohydrates: 44 g | Fiber: 3 g | Sodium: 52 mg

Creativity TWIST: Add dried cranberries + slivered almonds for a fall/holiday version (add carbs accordingly). Stir in 1 cup chickpeas for a vegetarian protein boost. Replace mushrooms with asparagus for spring flavor.

Oven Roasted Broccoli with Parmesan

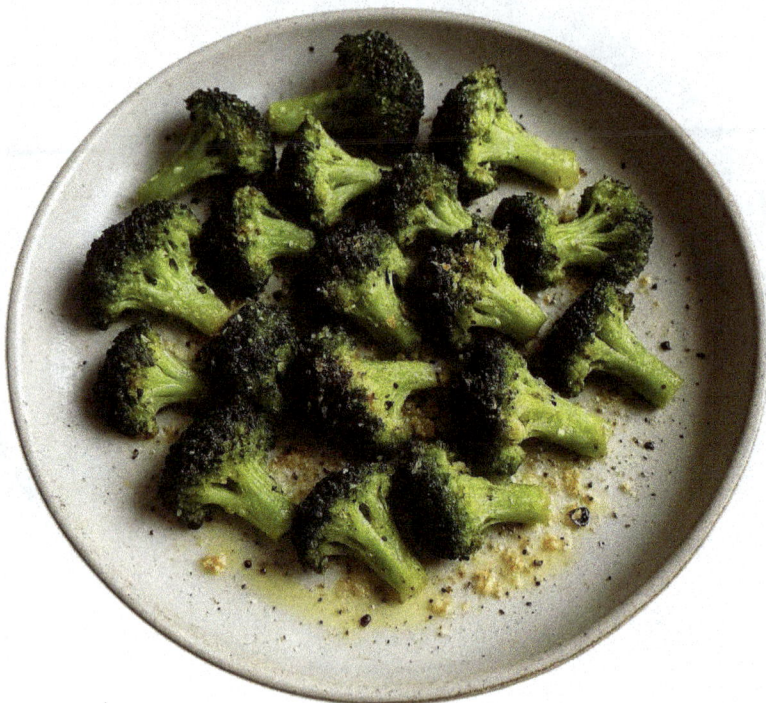

Servings 6 **Prep Time** 10' **Cook time** 20'

COST PER RECIPE $6 **GL** 2/ LOW

About this Recipe
Crisp-tender broccoli with Parmesan and lemon delivers bright, savory flavor that feels fresh and satisfying.

INGREDIENTS

- **6 cups broccoli florets (fresh or frozen, thawed)**
- • **2 tbsp olive oil**
- • **¼ cup grated Parmesan cheese**
- • **1 tbsp lemon juice**
- • **1 tsp garlic powder (seasoning — counts as 1 ingredient but not toward cost)**
- **Optional: black pepper, red pepper flakes, paprika**

DIRECTIONS

1. **Preheat oven to 400°F (204°C).**
2. **Toss broccoli with olive oil, garlic powder, and lemon juice.**
3. **Spread evenly on a baking sheet.**
4. **Roast 20 minutes, stirring halfway through.**
5. **Remove from oven and sprinkle Parmesan evenly over broccoli before serving.**

NUTRITION (1 CUP EACH)
Calories: 141 kcal | Protein: 5 g | Fat: 6 g | Carbohydrates: 7 g | Fiber: 4 g | Sodium: 90 mg

Creativity TWIST: Swap lemon juice for balsamic vinegar to add sweetness, or sprinkle with 2 tbsp slivered almonds after roasting for crunch and healthy fats.

Zesty Roasted Asparagus with Lemon

About this Recipe
Bright lemon and peppered asparagus roast to crisp-tender perfection, tasting fresh, vibrant, and satisfying.

INGREDIENTS

- **6 cups asparagus spears, trimmed**
- **2 tbsp olive oil**
- **1 tbsp lemon juice**
- **1 tsp lemon zest**
- **1 tsp black pepper (counts as an ingredient — seasonings not counted toward cost)**
- **Optional: garlic powder, red pepper flakes**

DIRECTIONS

1. Preheat oven to 400°F (204°C).
2. Toss asparagus with olive oil, lemon juice, lemon zest, and black pepper.
3. Spread evenly on a baking sheet.
4. Roast 12–15 minutes or until tender with light browning.

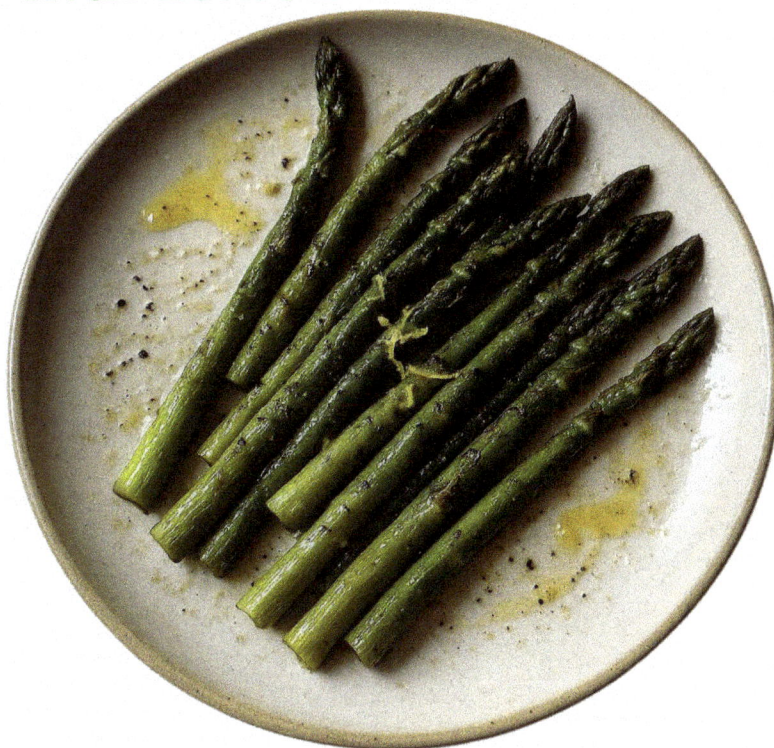

Servings	Prep Time	Cook time
6	8'	15'

GL	COST PER RECIPE
15/ MID	$5

NUTRITION (1 CUP EACH)
Calories: 92 kcal | Protein: 4 g | Fat: 6 g | Carbohydrates: 7 g | Fiber: 3 g | Sodium: 19 mg

Creativity TWIST: Swap lemon for balsamic glaze for a deeper flavor, or sprinkle with 2 tbsp Parmesan before serving for a kid-friendly version without a major sodium increase.

Roasted Green Beans & Tomatoes

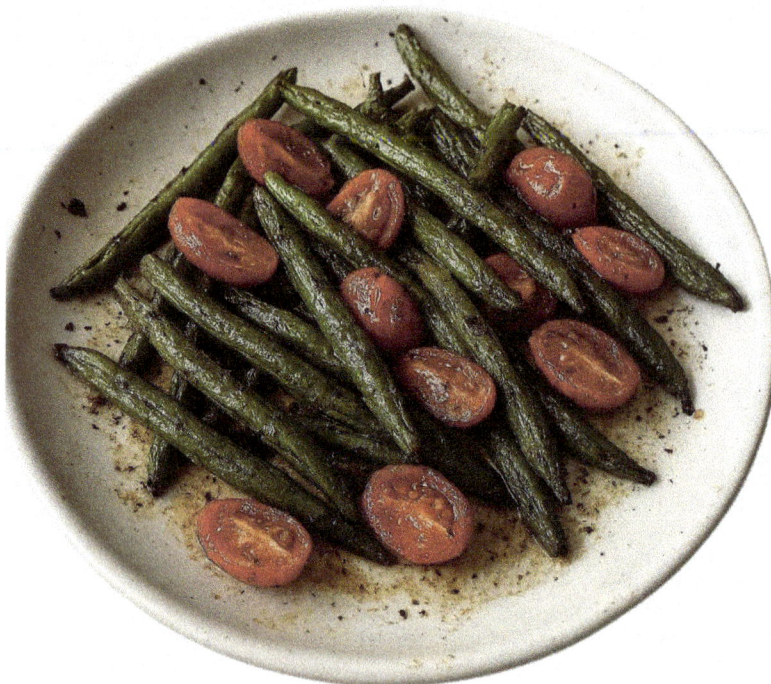

About this Recipe

Roasted green beans and juicy tomatoes offer a bright, savory bite that feels fresh, light, and satisfying.

INGREDIENTS

- 4 cups fresh green beans, trimmed
- 2 cups grape tomatoes, halved
- 2 tbsp olive oil
- 1 tsp balsamic vinegar
- 1 tsp Italian seasoning (seasoning — does not count toward cost)
- Optional: black pepper, garlic powder, parsley

Servings: **6** Prep Time: **8'** Cook time: **20'**

Cost per recipe: **$6** GL: **3/ LOW**

DIRECTIONS

1. Preheat oven to 400°F (204°C).
2. Toss green beans and tomatoes with olive oil, balsamic vinegar, and Italian seasoning.
3. Spread evenly on a baking sheet.
4. Roast 20 minutes, stirring halfway through.

NUTRITION (1 CUP EACH)
Calories: 80 kcal | Protein: 2 g | Fat: 5 g | Carbohydrates: 8 g | Fiber: 3 g | Sodium: 30 mg

Creativity TWIST: Top with 2 tbsp crumbled feta per family serving for a Mediterranean variation (adds sodium, so optional). Or sprinkle 1 tbsp pine nuts or slivered almonds right before serving for crunch and healthy fats.

Country Oven Roasted Cauliflower

> **About this Recipe**
>
> **Golden-roasted cauliflower steaks deliver smoky, savory flavor with a tender center and crisp edges.**

INGREDIENTS

- 2 large heads of cauliflower
- 3 tbsp olive oil
- 1 tbsp lemon juice
- 1 tsp garlic powder
- 1 tsp smoked paprika (counts as ingredient — not toward cost)
- Optional: black pepper, parsley, red pepper flakes

DIRECTIONS

1. Preheat oven to 425°F (218°C).
2. Remove outer leaves from cauliflower; slice each head into 3 thick "steaks."
3. Brush both sides with olive oil + lemon juice + garlic powder + paprika.
4. Place on a baking sheet and roast for 25 minutes, flipping halfway.

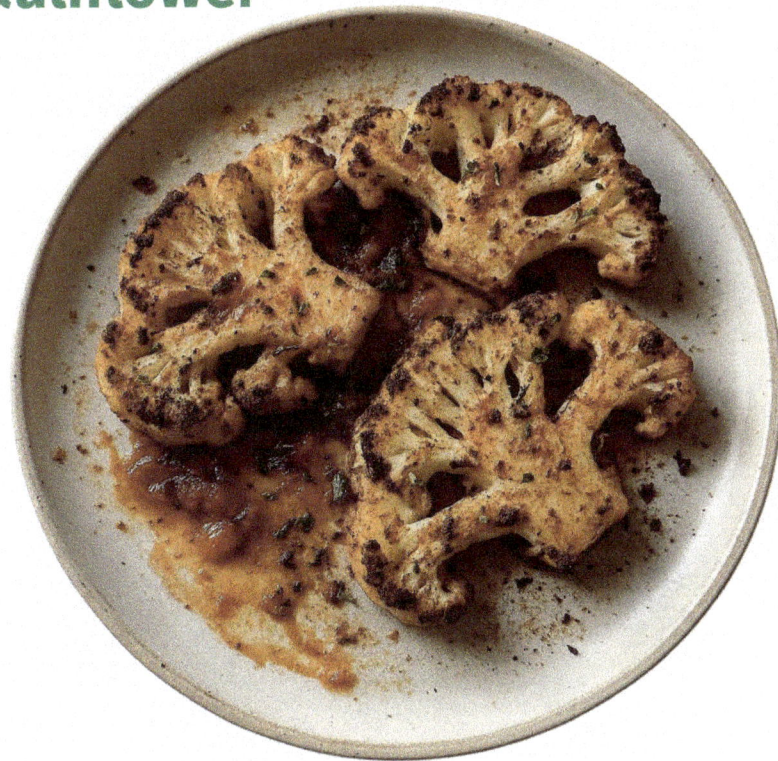

Servings	Prep Time	Cook time
6	10'	25'

GL	COST PER RECIPE
3/ LOW	$6

NUTRITION (1 STEAK EACH)
Calories: 92 kcal | Protein: 4 g | Fat: 6 g | Carbohydrates: 7 g | Fiber: 3 g | Sodium: 19 mg

Creativity TWIST: Add 1 tbsp grated Parmesan per steak after roasting for an elevated version, or top with a squeeze of fresh lemon + parsley for a bright finish.

Crispy Roasted Sweet Potatoes

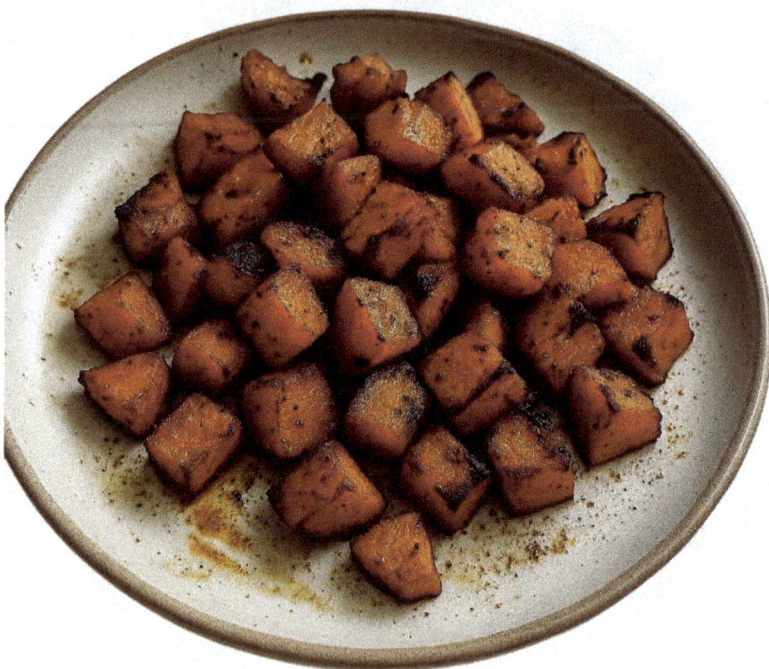

About this Recipe
Crispy-edged, tender-centered sweet potatoes taste lightly sweet and spiced, feeling warm, comforting, and satisfying.

INGREDIENTS

- 6 cups sweet potatoes, peeled or skin-on, diced into 1-inch cubes
- 2 tbsp olive oil
- 1 tbsp maple syrup (sugar-free optional)
- 1 tsp cinnamon
- 1 tsp black pepper (counts as ingredient — spices not counted toward cost)
- Optional: garlic powder, smoked paprika, nutmeg

Servings	Prep Time	Cook time
6	10'	30'

COST PER RECIPE	GL
$5	24/ HIGH

NUTRITION (1 CUP EACH)
Calories: 215 kcal | Protein: 3 g | Fat: 4 g | Carbohydrates: 41 g | Fiber: 4 g | Sodium: 27 mg

DIRECTIONS

1. Preheat oven to 400°F (204°C).
2. Toss sweet potato cubes with olive oil, maple syrup, cinnamon, and pepper.
3. Spread evenly on a parchment-lined baking sheet.
4. Roast 28–30 minutes, stirring halfway through for even browning.
5. Serving size = 1 cup

Creativity TWIST: Add ½ cup pecans near the end of roasting for crunch and healthy fats (adds ~2 g carbs per serving). For a savory version, skip the maple + cinnamon and replace with garlic powder + rosemary great with poultry.

Fresh Garden Green Salad

About this Recipe

Crisp, colorful vegetables deliver a fresh, crunchy salad that feels light, refreshing, and perfectly balanced.

INGREDIENTS

- **6 cups mixed salad greens (spinach, romaine, or spring mix)**
- **1 cup sliced cucumbers**
- **1 cup cherry tomatoes, halved**
- **¼ cup red onion, thinly sliced**
- **½ cup shredded carrots**
- **Optional seasonings: black pepper, parsley, lemon juice**

Serve with 2 tbsp dressing per serving (light Caesar, light ranch, or oil-free vinaigrette — added at the table to control calories and sodium).

DIRECTIONS

1. Add salad greens to a large bowl.
2. Top with cucumbers, tomatoes, red onion, and shredded carrots.
3. Toss gently just before serving.
4. Divide into 4 servings (about 1½ cups each).
5. Add dressing individually at the table.

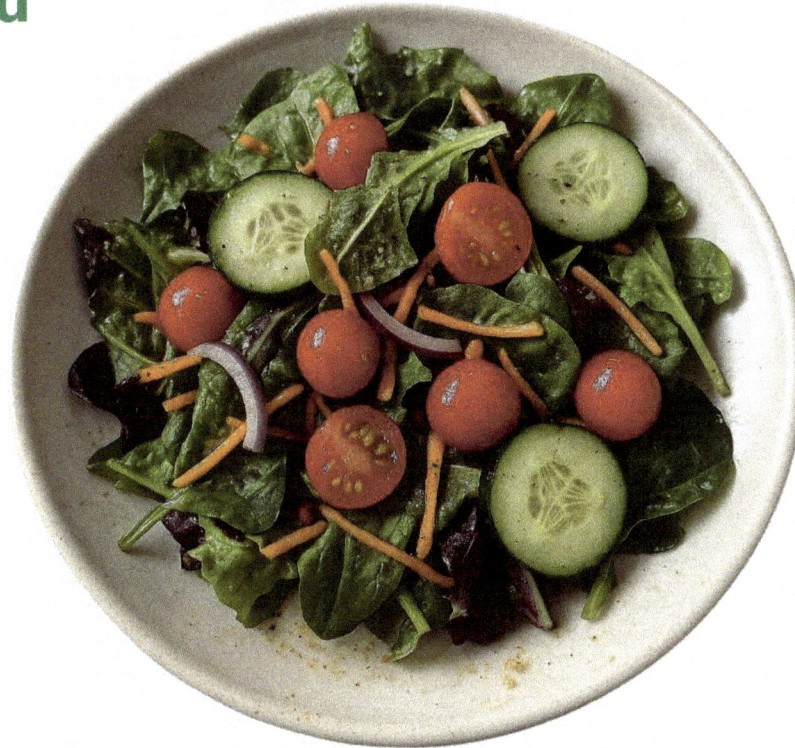

Servings **4**

Prep Time **8'**

Cook time **0'**

GL **2/ LOW**

COST PER RECIPE **$6**

NUTRITION (1½ CUPS PER SERVING)
Calories: 52 kcal | Protein: 2 g | Fat: 0 g | Carbohydrates: 7 g | Fiber: 3 g | Sodium: 19 mg

Creativity TWIST: Add ¼ cup chickpeas or edamame per serving to turn this into a high-protein lunch salad while keeping carbs controlled.

Savory Garlic Sautéed Mushrooms

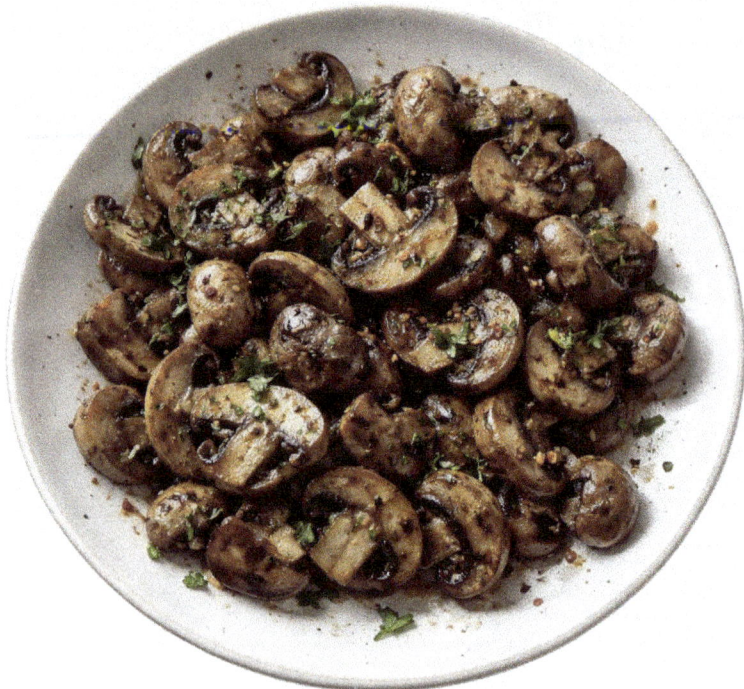

Servings 4

Prep Time 5'

Cook time 10'

COST PER RECIPE $3

GL 2/ LOW

NUTRITION (PER ½-CUP SERVING)
Calories: 78 kcal | Protein: 3 g | Fat: 5 g | Carbohydrates: 6 g | Fiber: 1 g | Sodium: 14 mg

Creativity TWIST: Stir in 1 tbsp balsamic vinegar during the final 2 minutes of cooking for rich depth of flavor (no impact on GL) — or sprinkle 2 tbsp shaved parmesan on top for savoriness without significantly raising carbs.

About this Recipe

Savory garlic mushrooms cook to tender perfection, delivering rich umami flavor that feels warm and comforting.

INGREDIENTS

- 4 cups sliced mushrooms (white or baby bella)
- • 1 tbsp olive oil
- • 1 tbsp minced garlic
- • ¼ tsp black pepper
- • 2 tbsp chopped fresh parsley (optional)
- Optional seasonings (NOT counted): red pepper flakes, garlic powder, onion powder

DIRECTIONS

1. Heat olive oil in a large skillet over medium heat.
2. Add mushrooms and sauté 6–7 minutes, stirring occasionally.
3. Add minced garlic and black pepper; cook 2–3 more minutes until tender and browned.
4. Remove from heat and stir in parsley if desired.

Crispy Oven Roasted Summer Squash

About this Recipe

Lightly crisped summer squash tastes fresh and garlicky, feeling light, satisfying, and effortlessly delicious.

INGREDIENTS

- 2 cups sliced yellow summer squash
- 2 cups sliced zucchini
- 1 tbsp olive oil
- 1 tsp minced garlic
- ¼ tsp black pepper

Optional (NOT counted): ¼ tsp dried Italian seasoning, lemon zest, basil

DIRECTIONS

1. Preheat oven to 400°F (205°C).
2. Add squash and zucchini to a large bowl.
3. Toss with olive oil, garlic, black pepper, and Italian seasoning if using.
4. Spread evenly on a parchment-lined baking sheet.
5. Roast 18–20 minutes, flipping halfway through, until tender and lightly golden.

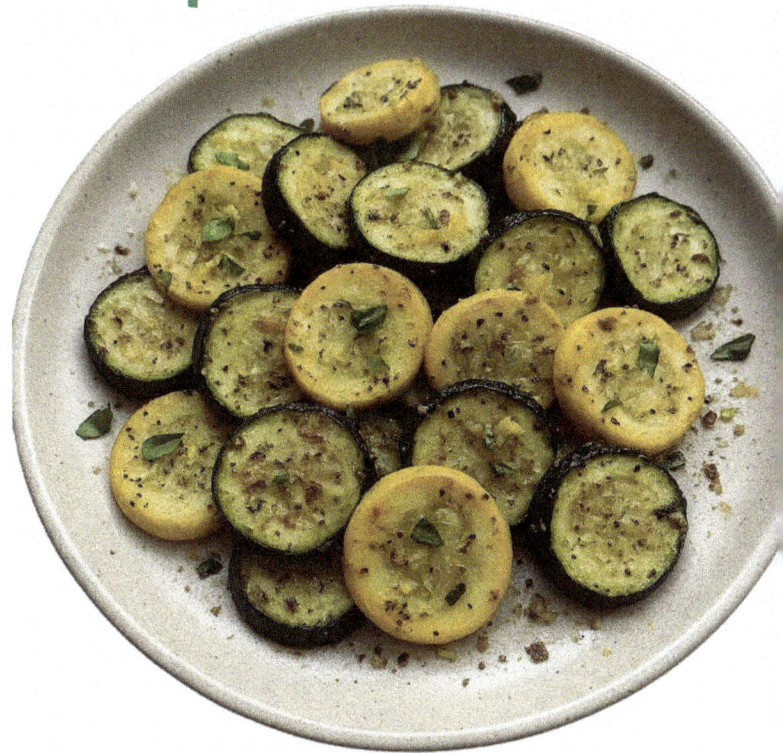

Servings 4 | Prep Time 8' | Cook time 20'

GL 3/ LOW | COST PER RECIPE $3

NUTRITION (½ CUP EACH)

Calories: 52 kcal | Protein: 2 g | Fat: 0 g | Carbohydrates: 7 g | Fiber: 3 g | Sodium: 19 mg

Creativity TWIST: Italian version: sprinkle 2 tbsp grated Parmesan during the last 5 minutes of roasting. Mediterranean version: add fresh basil + lemon zest right before serving.

Carmelized Oven Roasted Carrots

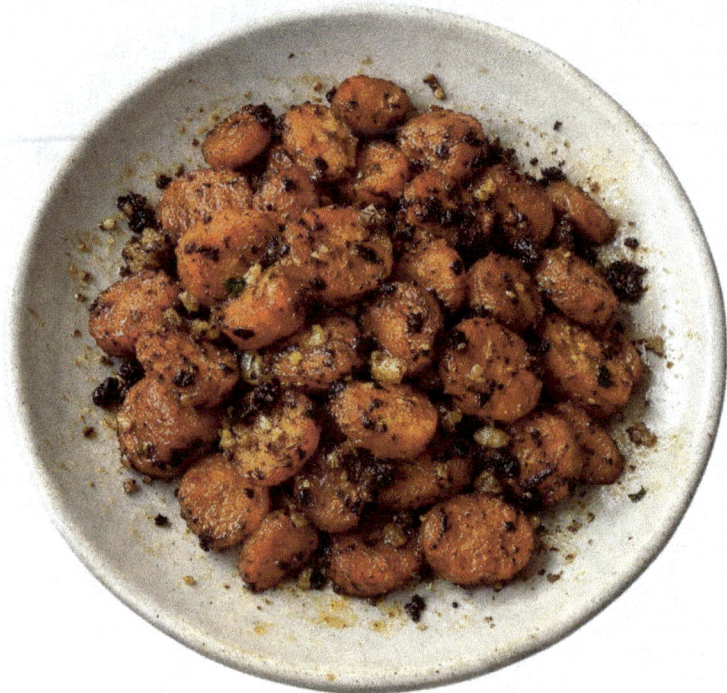

About this Recipe
Naturally sweet carrots caramelize beautifully, delivering a warm, savory-sweet bite that feels comforting and satisfying.

INGREDIENTS

- **3 cups sliced carrots (fresh or frozen)**
- **1 tbsp olive oil**
- **1 tsp minced garlic**
- **¼ tsp black pepper**
- **½ tsp dried parsley (optional)**
- **Optional seasonings (NOT counted): smoked paprika, thyme, cinnamonr**

Servings	Prep Time	Cook time
4	8'	22'

COST PER RECIPE	GL
$2	8/ LOW

DIRECTIONS

1. Preheat oven to 400°F (205°C)
2. Place sliced carrots in a bowl and toss with olive oil, garlic, black pepper, and parsley if using
3. Spread evenly on a parchment-lined baking sheet
4. Roast 20–22 minutes, stirring halfway through, until edges are lightly browned and carrots are fork-tender.

NUTRITION (½ CUP EACH)
Calories: 82 kcal | Protein: 1 g | Fat: 5 g | Carbohydrates: 10 g | Fiber: 3 g | Sodium: 41 mg

Creativity TWIST: Add 1 tbsp balsamic vinegar during the last 5 minutes of roasting for a tangy-sweet finish without increasing GL or sprinkle with ½ tsp smoked paprika for a warm, savory flavor

Cozy Spinach-Parmesan Orzo Skillet

About this Recipe
Tender orzo with wilted spinach and Parmesan creates a cozy, savory skillet that feels comforting and satisfying.

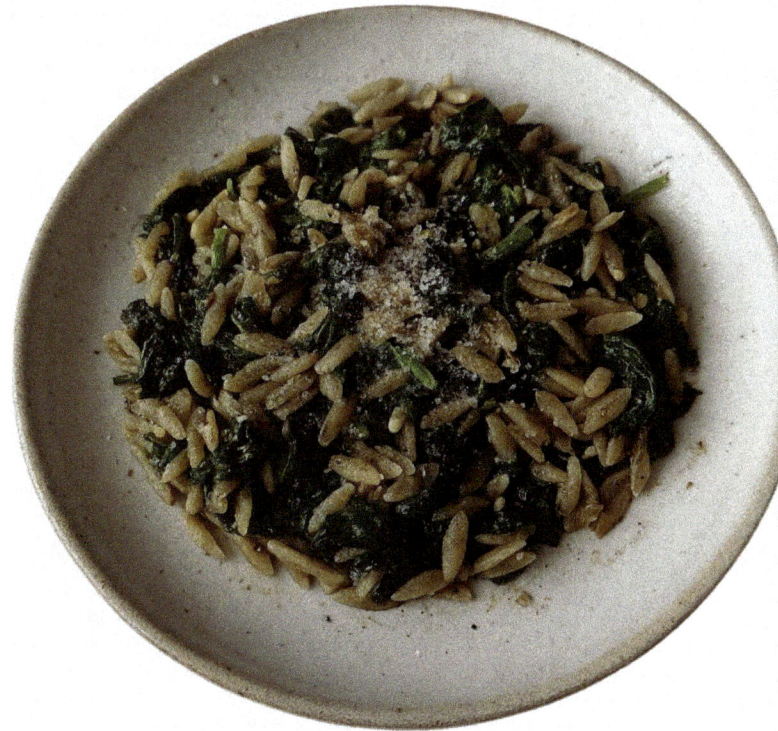

INGREDIENTS

- 1 cup whole-grain orzo
- 2 cups fresh spinach, chopped
- 1 tbsp olive oil
- 2 tbsp grated parmesan cheese
- ¼ tsp black pepper

Optional seasonings (NOT counted): lemon zest, parsley, crushed red pepper

DIRECTIONS

1. Bring 4 cups of water to a boil and cook whole-grain orzo according to package directions (9–10 minutes).
2. Drain well and return to the pot.
3. Stir in olive oil and black pepper.
4. Add chopped spinach and mix until wilted from the heat of the pasta.
5. Sprinkle with parmesan and divide into 4 servings (½ cup each).

Servings	Prep Time	Cook time
4	8'	12'

GL	COST PER RECIPE
18/ MID	$4

NUTRITION (½ CUP EACH)
Calories: 168 kcal | Protein: 6 g | Fat: 6 g | Carbohydrates: 23 g | Fiber: 2 g | Sodium: 61 mg

Creativity TWIST: Add lemon zest + parsley for a bright Mediterranean flavor Swap spinach for arugula for a peppery version.

Creamy Cheesy Broccoli Couscous

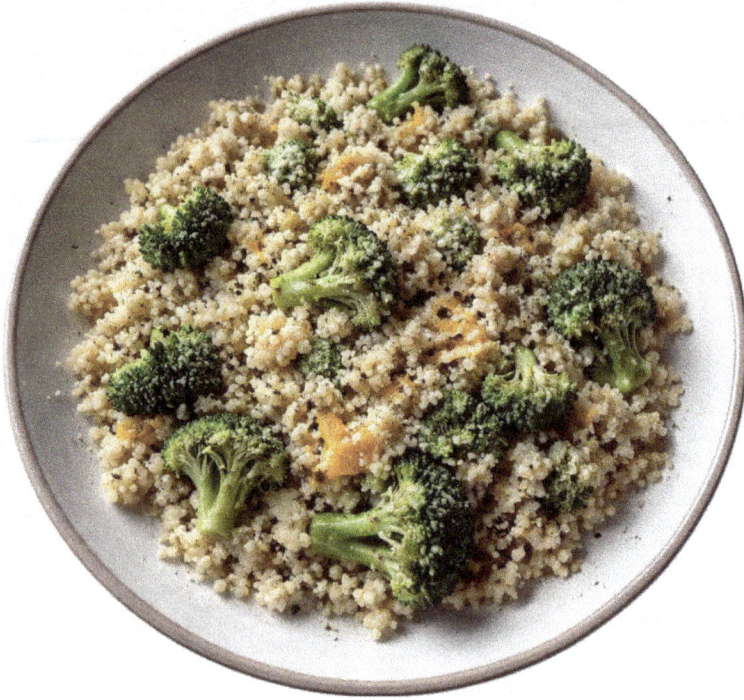

Servings	Prep Time	Cook time
4	10'	8'

COST PER RECIPE	GL
$4	20/ HIGH

NUTRITION (½ CUP EACH)
Calories: 182 kcal | Protein: 8 g | Fat: 6 g | Carbohydrates: 21 g | Fiber: 3 g | Sodium: 154 mg

Creativity TWIST: Mediterranean style: swap cheddar for 2 tbsp crumbled feta + lemon zest.
Kid-friendly version: use mild cheddar + finely chopped broccoli

About this Recipe
Fluffy couscous and melty cheese wrap tender broccoli in a savory, comforting bite that feels wholesome.

INGREDIENTS

- **1 cup whole-wheat couscous**
- **2 cups chopped broccoli (fresh or frozen)**
- **½ cup reduced-fat shredded cheddar cheese**
- **1 tbsp olive oil**
- **¼ tsp black pepper**
- **Optional seasonings (NOT counted): lemon zest, parsley, garlic powder**

DIRECTIONS

1. **Bring 1 cup water + 1 cup low-sodium broth (or water only) to a boil**
2. **Stir in couscous, cover, and remove from heat; let sit for 5 minutes**
3. **Steam broccoli for 4 minutes (microwave or stovetop) until tender**
4. **Fluff couscous with a fork; stir in olive oil and black pepper**
5. **Fold in broccoli, then sprinkle in shredded cheddar until lightly melted.**

Rustic Toasted Ravioli and Veggies

About this Recipe
Crispy baked ravioli and tender vegetables create a rustic, comforting dish with a satisfying crunch and cozy flavor.

INGREDIENTS

- 1 (12 oz) bag frozen whole-wheat cheese ravioli
- 2 cups frozen mixed vegetables, thawed or lightly steamed
- 1 cup whole-wheat breadcrumbs
- ½ cup low-fat shredded Parmesan and mozzarella blend
- 2 eggs, beaten
- ½ tsp black pepper

Servings 4 | Prep Time 12' | Cook time 12'

GL 20/HIGH | COST PER RECIPE $10

DIRECTIONS

1. Preheat oven to 425°F (218°C) and line a baking sheet with parchment paper.
2. Dip each frozen ravioli into beaten egg, then coat in whole-wheat breadcrumbs.
3. Place ravioli in a single layer on the baking sheet and sprinkle with black pepper.
4. Bake 10–12 minutes, turning halfway through.
5. During the last 2 minutes of baking, sprinkle shredded cheese evenly on top.
6. While ravioli is baked, warm or steam mixed vegetables.
7. Serve 4 ravioli with ½ cup of vegetables per serving.

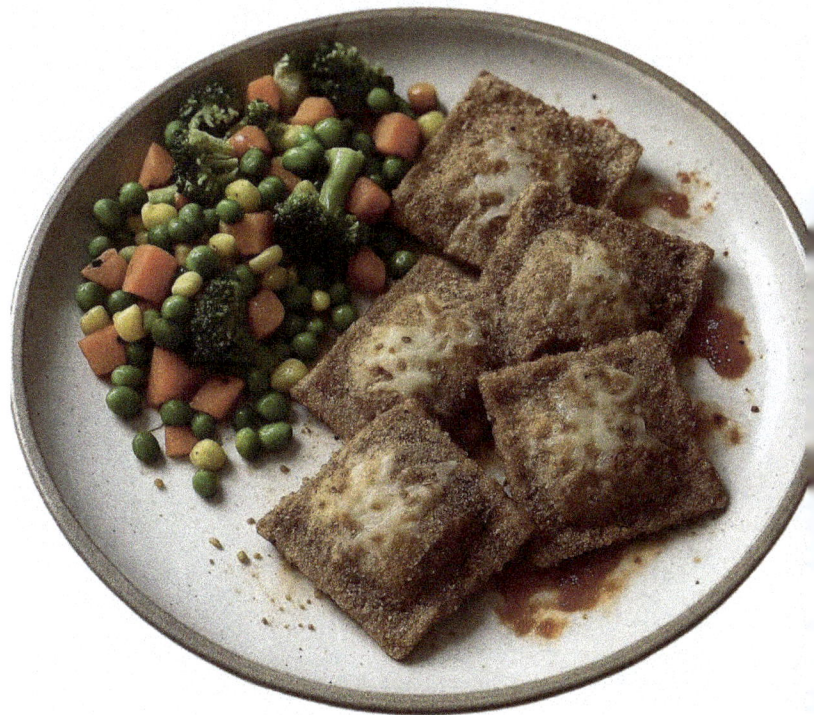

NUTRITION 4 RAVIOLI +1/2 CUP VEG.
Calories: 370 kcal | Protein: 20 g | Fat: 10 g | Carbohydrates: 48 g | Fiber: 4 g | Sodium: 500 mg

Creativity TWIST: Serve vegetables mixed into the breadcrumb coating for extra crunch, or mix ½ cup steamed spinach into the ravioli before baking for a richer texture without adding sodium.

Cozy Black Bean & Corn Quesadillas

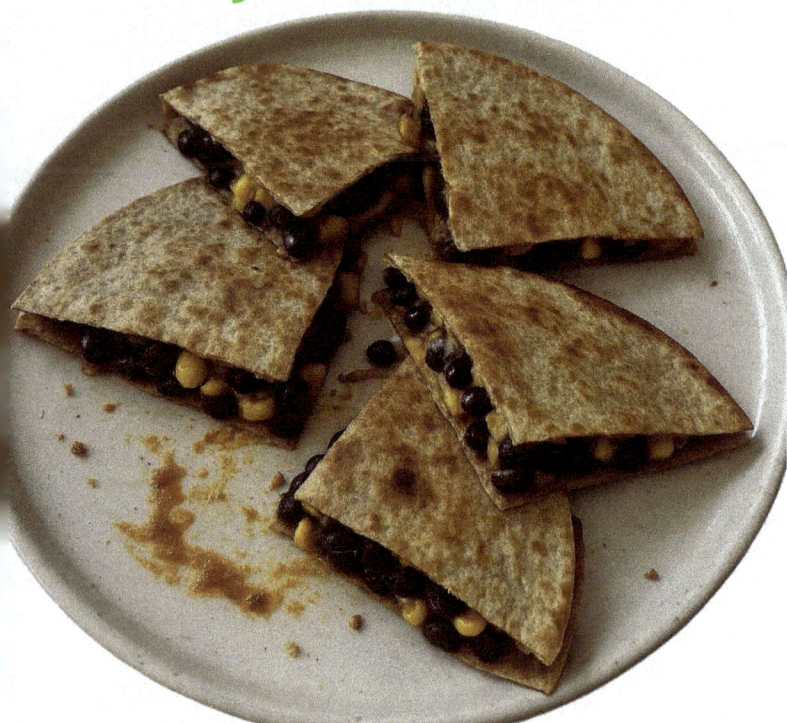

About this Recipe
Warm, cheesy quesadillas with hearty beans and corn deliver cozy flavor, satisfying crunch, and comforting fullness.

Servings: 4
Prep Time: 8'
Cook time: 8'
COST PER RECIPE: $5
GL: 15/ MID

INGREDIENTS

- 1 can (15 oz) black beans, rinsed and drained
- 1 cup frozen corn (thawed)
- 1 cup reduced-fat shredded Mexican blend cheese
- 2 tsp no-salt taco seasoning
- 8 small whole-wheat tortillas (2 per serving)

DIRECTIONS

1. In a bowl, combine black beans, corn, cheese, and taco seasoning.
2. Divide filling evenly across 8 tortillas and fold each in half.
3. Heat a non-stick skillet over medium heat.
4. Cook quesadillas 2–3 minutes per side until browned and cheese is melted.
5. Slice and serve warm.

NUTRITION 1 QUESADILLAS
Calories: 230 | Protein: 11 g | Fat: 10 g | Carbohydrates: 32 g | Fiber: 6 g | Sodium: 289 mg

Creativity TWIST: Add chopped cilantro and a squeeze of lime juice before serving to boost flavor without increasing sodium. To increase protein, top with 2 tbsp non-fat Greek yogurt instead of sour cream.

Hearty Homestyle Vegetable Chili

About this Recipe

Slow-simmered beans and vegetables create a hearty chili with bold flavor that feels warm and deeply satisfying.

INGREDIENTS

- 1 can (15 oz) low-sodium black beans, rinsed and drained
- 1 can (15 oz) low-sodium kidney beans, rinsed and drained
- 1 can (15 oz) diced tomatoes (no salt added)
- 2 cups of mixed vegetables (bell pepper, onion, corn, zucchini)
- 2 tbsp chili powder (no-salt blend)

DIRECTIONS

1. Add all ingredients to a large pot.
2. Stir well and bring to a simmer over medium heat.
3. Reduce the heat and cook for 30 minutes, stirring occasionally.
4. Serve hot. Add water if you prefer a thinner consistency.

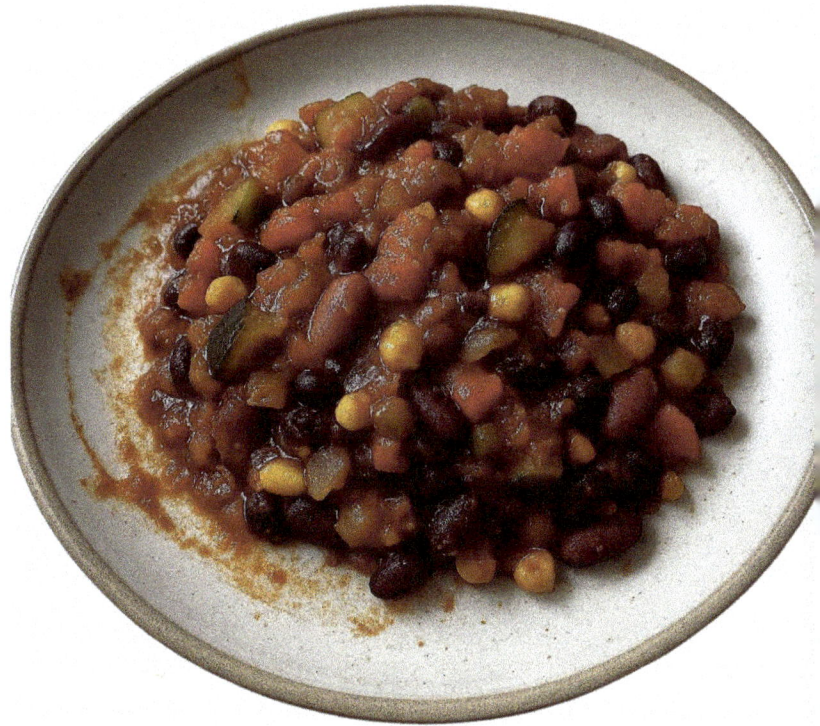

Servings 4 | Prep Time 10' | Cook time 30'

GL 14/ MID | COST PER RECIPE $6

NUTRITION (1 CUP)
Calories: 250 | Protein: 14 g | Fat: 2 g | Carbohydrates: 47 g | Fiber: 13 g | Sodium: 14 mg

Creativity TWIST: Add sliced avocado on top for creaminess (adds healthy fat without raising sodium) or 1 tbsp Greek yogurt for a chili "sour cream" effect with added protein.

Hearty Veggie Enchilada Bake

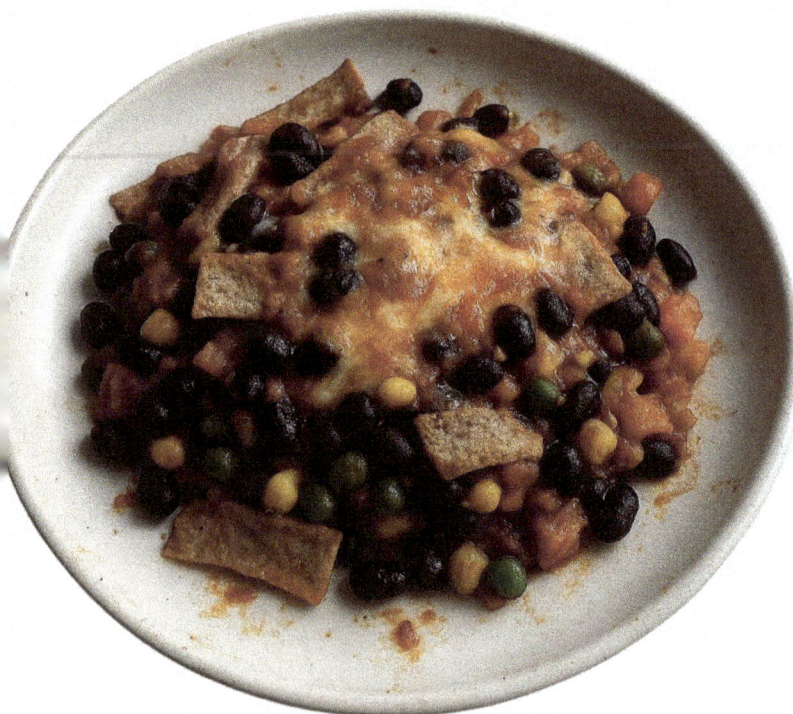

Servings	Prep Time	Cook time
4	12'	22'

COST PER RECIPE	GL
$8	17/ MID

NUTRITION (1¼ CUPS PER SERVING)
Calories: 398 kcal | Protein: 27 g | Fat: 7 g | Carbohydrates: 47 g | Fiber: 11 g | Sodium: 289 mg

Creativity TWIST: Add ¼ cup non-fat Greek yogurt on top for creaminess without sodium, or swap black beans for pinto beans for a milder flavor profile with the same nutrition.

About this Recipe
Layers of veggies, beans, and melty cheese bake into a cozy enchilada dish that feels hearty and comforting.

INGREDIENTS

- 1 (15 oz) can black beans, rinsed and drained
- 3 cups mixed vegetables (fresh or frozen)
- 6 small whole-wheat tortillas, cut into strips
- 1 cup no-salt-added tomato sauce
- 1 cup reduced-fat shredded Mexican-blend cheese

DIRECTIONS

1. Preheat oven to 375°F (190°C).
2. In a large mixing bowl, combine black beans, mixed vegetables, tomato sauce, and ½ cup shredded cheese.
3. Add tortilla strips and stir until fully coated.
4. Spread mixture into a baking dish and top with remaining ½ cup cheese.
5. Bake 20–22 minutes, or until hot and cheese is melted.
6. Cool 5 minutes before serving (1¼ cups per serving).

Cozy Chickpea & Spinach Skillet Meal

About this Recipe
Tender chickpeas, spinach, and melted cheese come together in a cozy skillet that feels hearty and comforting.

INGREDIENTS

- **2 (15 oz) cans chickpeas, rinsed and drained**
- **3 cups fresh spinach, chopped**
- **1 cup no-salt-added tomato sauce**
- **1 cup reduced-fat shredded mozzarella**
- **1 cup frozen mixed vegetables**

Optional seasonings (NOT counted): minced garlic, black pepper, Italian seasoning, crushed red pepper

DIRECTIONS

1. Spray a large skillet with cooking spray (no cost added) and warm over medium heat.
2. Add chickpeas and optional garlic; cook 2–3 minutes.
3. Add tomato sauce and mixed vegetables; simmer 5 minutes, stirring occasionally.
4. Stir in chopped spinach and cook 2–3 minutes until wilted.
5. Top with mozzarella and cook for 2 minutes covered to melt.
6. Serve warm (1¼ cups per serving).

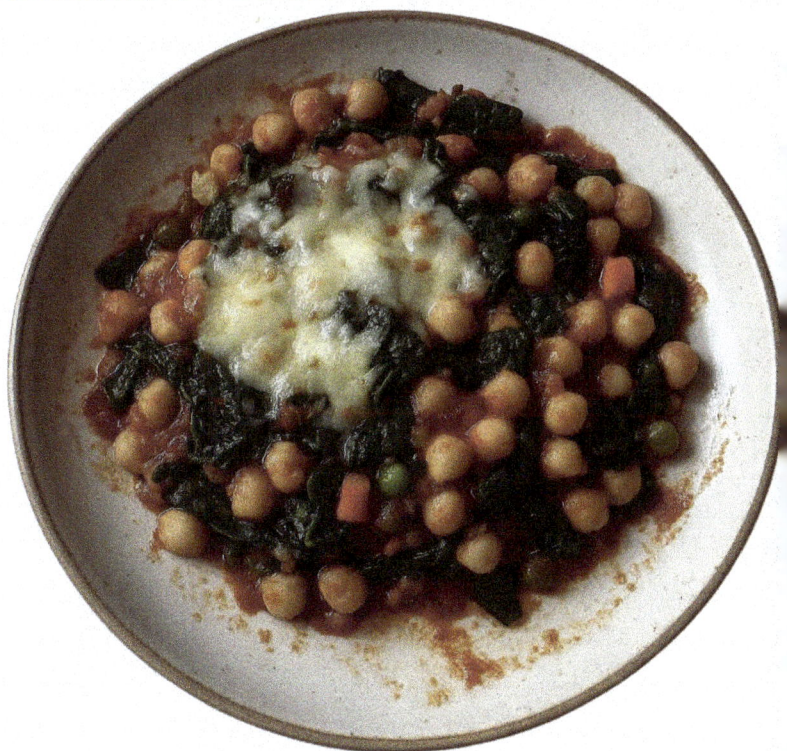

Servings	Prep Time	Cook time
4	8'	12'

GL	COST PER RECIPE
14/ MID	$8

NUTRITION (1¼ CUPS PER SERVING)
Calories: 358 kcal | Protein: 24 g | Fat: 5 g | Carbohydrates: 42 g | Fiber: 12 g | Sodium: 284 mg

Creativity TWIST: Swap mozzarella for feta to make a Greek-style version or serve over brown rice for higher-carb days (+17–22 g carbs per serving).

Sweet Savory Teriyaki Edamame Noodle Bowl

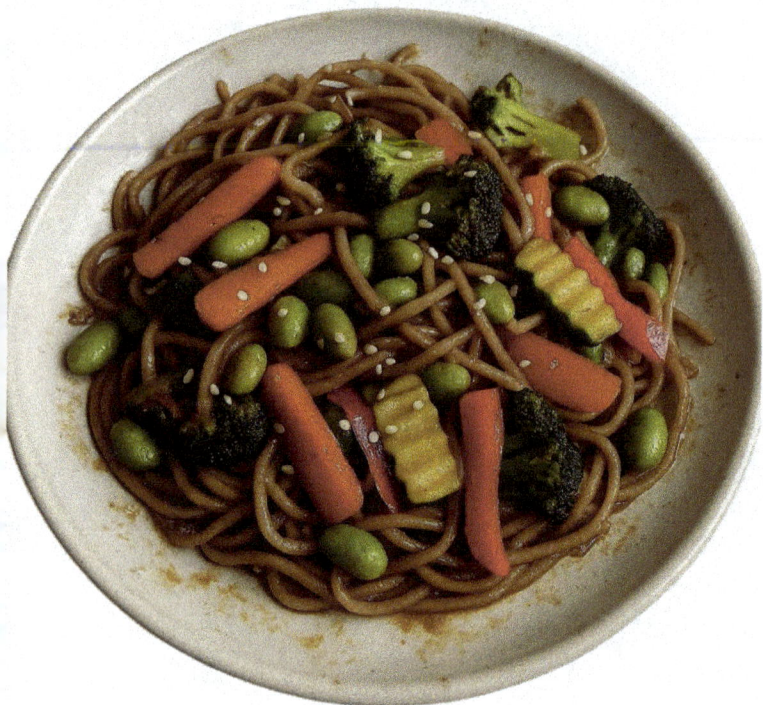

About this Recipe
Tender noodles, crisp vegetables, and edamame come together in a sweet-savory bowl that feels filling and flavorful.

INGREDIENTS

- **8 oz whole-grain noodles**
- **2 cups shelled edamame**
- **3 cups stir-fry vegetables (fresh or frozen)**
- **¼ cup low-sodium teriyaki sauce**
- **1 tbsp sesame seeds**

Optional seasonings (NOT counted): minced garlic, black pepper, green onion

Servings	Prep Time	Cook time
4	10'	12'

COST PER RECIPE	GL
$10	22/ HIGH

DIRECTIONS

1. Cook whole-grain noodles according to package directions; drain and set aside.
2. Sauté stir-fry vegetables in a large skillet for 5–6 minutes.
3. Add edamame and optional garlic; cook 3 minutes.
4. Reduce the heat to low and stir in cooked noodles and teriyaki sauce; toss to coat.
5. Sprinkle sesame seeds on top and serve warm (about 1¼ cups per serving).

NUTRITION 1¼ CUPS PER SERVING
Calories: ~430 kcal | Protein: 26 g | Fat: 11 g | Carbohydrates: 56 g | Fiber: 11 g | Sodium: 279 mg

Creativity TWIST: Add chili paste for spice, or substitute whole-grain spaghetti for udon noodles to change the texture without altering the nutrition.

Cozy Edamame Rice Skillet

About this Recipe
Savory edamame and fluffy eggs cook into a cozy skillet that feels filling, comforting, and energizing.

INGREDIENTS

- 2 cups shelled edamame
- 1 (12 oz) bag of cauliflower rice
- 1 cup peas and carrots (fresh or frozen)
- 2 eggs, beaten
- 3 tbsp low-sodium soy sauce

Optional seasonings (NOT counted): black pepper, onion powder, sesame oil

DIRECTIONS

1. Warm a large skillet over medium-high heat, then cook the cauliflower rice with peas and carrots for 4–5 minutes.
2. Add edamame and cook 3 minutes.
3. Push the mixture to one side; pour beaten eggs on the empty side and scramble until fully cooked.
4. Combine everything and stir in soy sauce.

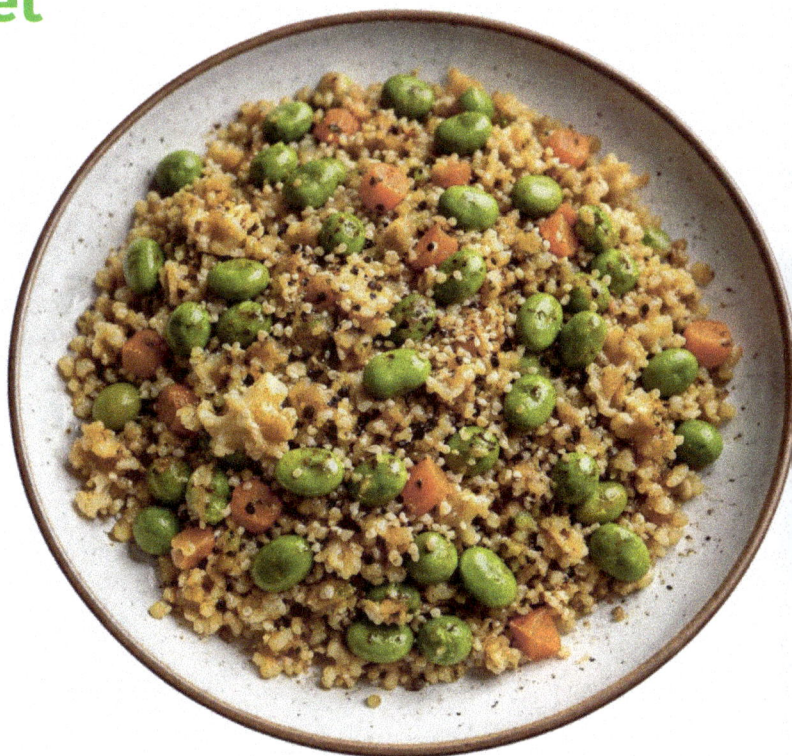

Servings **4** | Prep Time **5'** | Cook time **10'**

GL **18/ MID** | COST PER RECIPE **$9**

NUTRITION 1¼ CUPS PER SERVING
Calories: ~277 kcal | Protein: 18 g | Fat: 5 g | Carbohydrates: 46 g | Fiber: 9 g | Sodium: 69 mg

Creativity TWIST: Add a teaspoon of sesame oil for a toasted flavor, or serve with 1 cup brown rice on higher-carb days (+45 g carbs per serving).

Savory Edamame Noursish Bowl

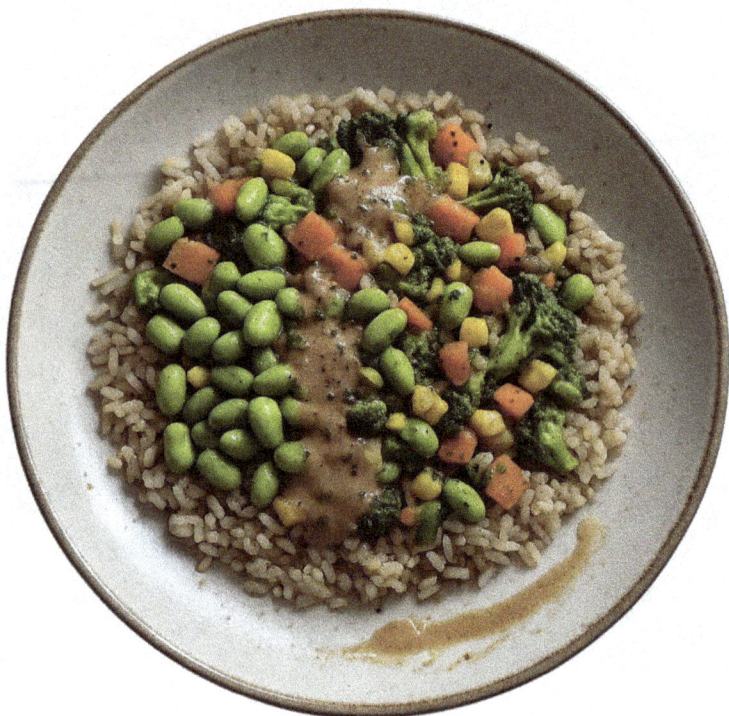

Servings	Prep Time	Cook time
4	15'	15'

COST PER RECIPE	GL
$7	22/ HIGH

About this Recipe
Savory edamame, hearty grains, and a creamy lemon-peanut drizzle create a filling, satisfying bowl.

INGREDIENTS

- 2 cups shelled edamame (frozen)
- 2 cups cooked brown rice (from 1 cup uncooked)
- 2 cups frozen mixed vegetables, thawed
- ¼ cup powdered peanut butter (PB2)
- 2 tbsp lemon juice

Optional seasonings (NOT counted): black pepper, garlic powder, parsley

DIRECTIONS

1. Spray a large non-stick skillet with cooking spray (no cost added).
2. Warm the edamame and thawed mixed vegetables over medium heat for 4–6 minutes
3. Add cooked brown rice and stir to combine.
4. In a small bowl, whisk PB2, lemon juice, and water until creamy, thinning as desired.
5. Divide into 4 bowls (1¼ cups each) and drizzle dressing over top just before serving.
6. Serve warm or chilled.

NUTRITION 1¼ CUPS PER SERVING
Calories: ~277 kcal | Protein: 18 g | Fat: 5 g | Carbohydrates: 46 g | Fiber: 9 g | Sodium: 69 mg

Creativity TWIST: Swap brown rice for whole-wheat pasta or add a cucumber for freshness while keeping the total cost under $10.

Creamy Parmesan Zucchini Carbonara

About this Recipe

Creamy egg-parmesan pasta with zucchini and peas delivers classic comfort with a fresh, satisfying twist.

INGREDIENTS

- 8 oz whole-wheat spaghetti
- 2 large eggs
- ½ cup grated parmesan cheese
- 2 cups shredded zucchini
- 2 cups frozen peas

Optional seasonings (NOT counted): black pepper (generous), garlic powder, crushed red pepper

DIRECTIONS

1. Cook whole-wheat spaghetti according to package directions; add peas during the last 2 minutes of boiling.
2. Meanwhile, sauté shredded zucchini in a dry skillet for 3–4 minutes to remove moisture (no oil needed).
3. Whisk eggs and parmesan together in a bowl.
4. Add pasta and peas to the skillet with zucchini OFF heat.
5. Pour the egg-parmesan mixture over the hot pasta and toss vigorously until a creamy sauce forms from residual heat.

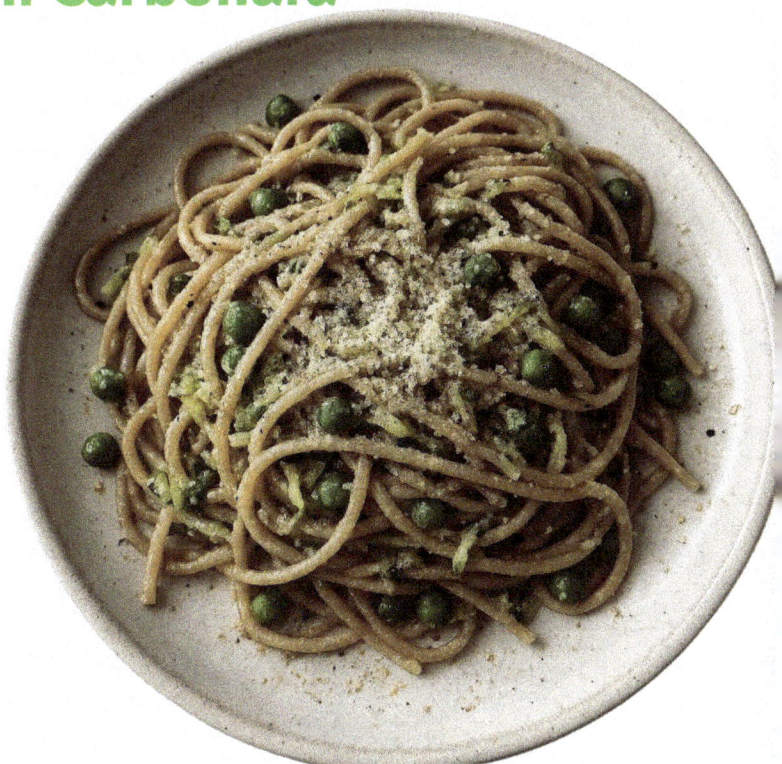

Servings **4** | Prep Time **10'** | Cook time **12'**

GL **15/ MID** | COST PER RECIPE **$8**

NUTRITION 1¼ CUPS PER SERVING
Calories: ~356 kcal | Protein: 20 g | Fat: 8 g | Carbohydrates: 53 g | Fiber: 8 g | Sodium: 265 mg

Creativity TWIST: Add lemon zest + freshly cracked black pepper for a restaurant-style finish. Swap peas for chopped asparagus in spring — no change to cost or nutrition

Buttery Soy-Garlic Linguine with Mushrooms & Edamame

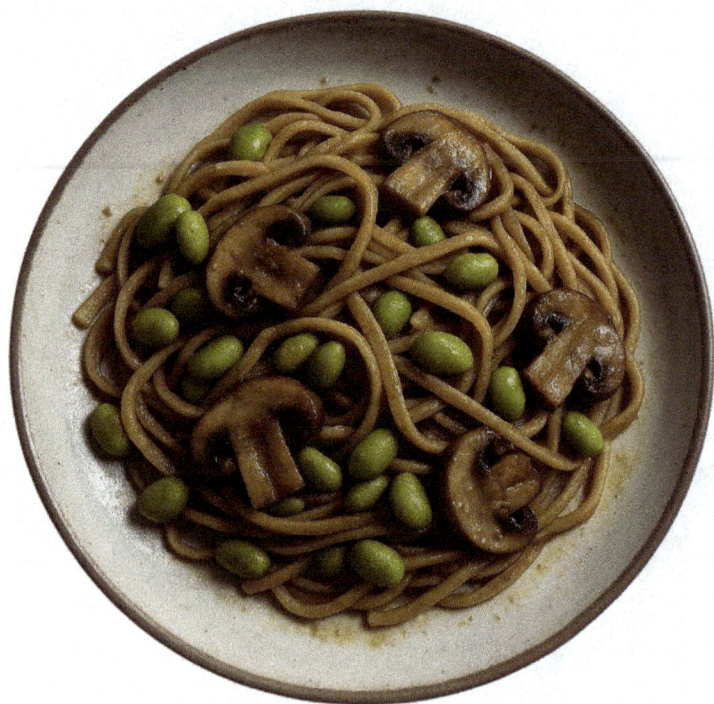

Servings	Prep Time	Cook time
4	10'	14'

COST PER RECIPE	GL
$10	18/ MID

NUTRITION 1¼ CUPS PER SERVING
Calories: ~315 kcal | Protein: 17 g | Fat: 8 g | Carbohydrates: 49 g | Fiber: 10 g | Sodium: ~341 mg

Creativity TWIST: Add sliced green onions and lemon zest for brightness — or swap linguine for soba noodles for even more protein.

About this Recipe
Tender linguine tossed with umami-rich mushrooms and edamame creates a savory, cozy pasta bowl.

INGREDIENTS

- 8 oz whole-grain linguine
- 2 cups sliced mushrooms
- 2 cups shelled edamame
- 2 tbsp light butter
- 2 tbsp low-sodium soy sauce

Optional seasonings (NOT counted): minced garlic, lemon zest, black pepper, crushed red pepper

DIRECTIONS

1. Cook linguine according to package directions; reserve ¼ cup pasta cooking water.
2. Sauté mushrooms in a large skillet for 5–6 minutes.
3. Add edamame and cook 3 minutes.
4. Turn the heat to low and stir in butter and soy sauce until melted.
5. Add linguine and a splash of pasta water and toss to coat.

Fiesta Chicken Quesadilla

About this Recipe
Bold taco-seasoned chicken and gooey cheese come together in a crispy quesadilla that feels hearty and comforting.

INGREDIENTS

- 2 cups cooked, shredded chicken breast
- 1 cup reduced-fat shredded Mexican blend cheese
- 2 tsp no-salt taco seasoning
- 8 small whole-wheat tortillas (2 per serving)
- 2 tsp olive oil (for cooking)

DIRECTIONS

1. In a bowl, mix shredded chicken and taco seasoning.
2. Sprinkle cheese onto 8 tortillas and top with seasoned chicken.
3. Fold each tortilla in half to form quesadillas.
4. Heat olive oil in a skillet over medium heat.
5. Cook each quesadilla 2–3 minutes per side, until lightly browned and the cheese is melted.
6. Slice and serve warm.

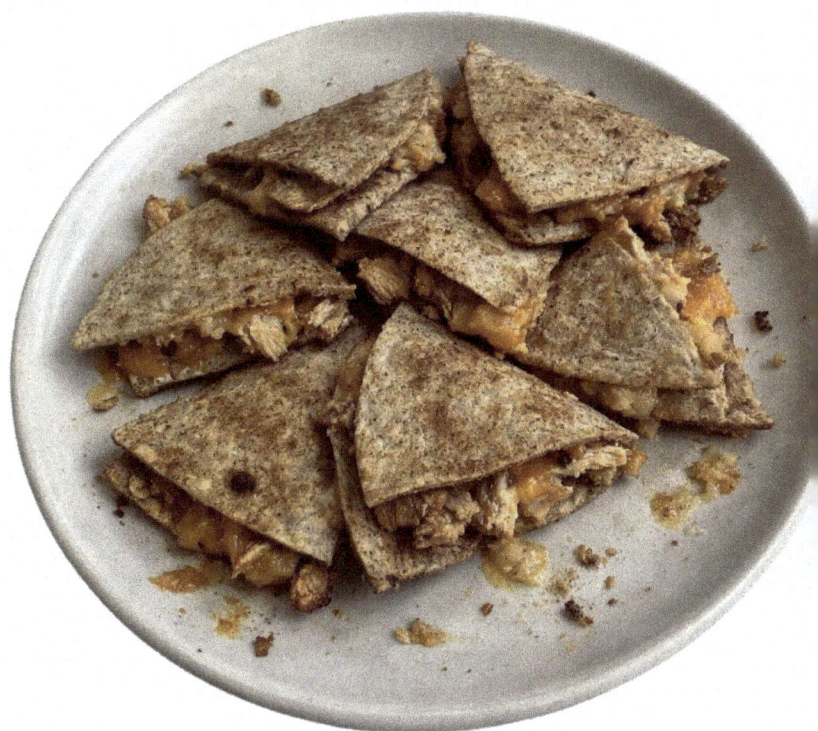

Servings	Prep Time	Cook time
4	10'	8'

GL	COST PER RECIPE
15/ MID	$7

NUTRITION 2 QUESADILLAS/ SERVING
Calories: 418 kcal | Protein: 32 g | Fat: 11 g | Carbohydrates: 44 g | Fiber: 6 g | Sodium: 361 mg

Creativity TWIST: Add fresh cilantro and lime before serving for bright flavor without added sodium. For higher fiber and protein, add ¼ cup black beans to the filling (+3 g carbs per serving).

Classic Tuna and Cheddar Melt

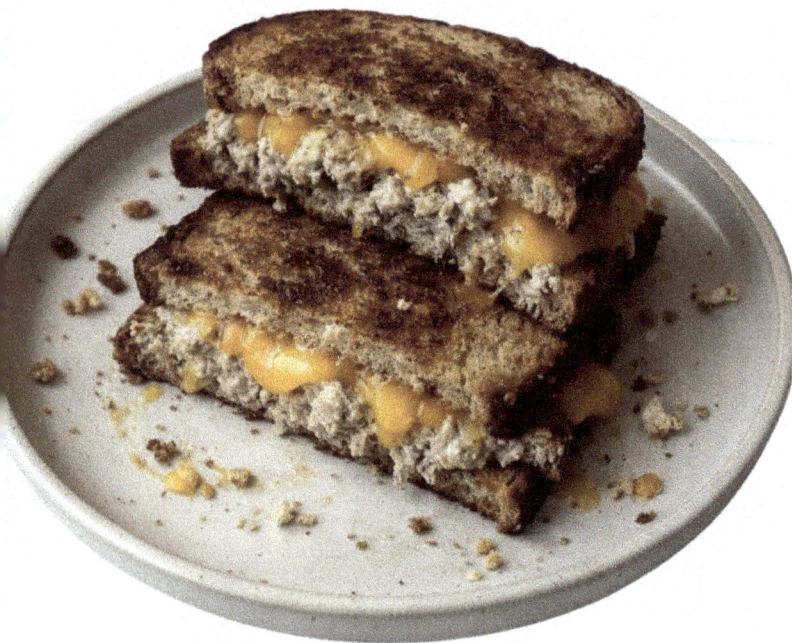

About this Recipe
Savory tuna blended smooth and topped with melted cheddar delivers a warm, nostalgic melt that satisfies.

INGREDIENTS

- 2 cans (5 oz each) of low-sodium tuna in water, drained
- ½ cup non-fat Greek yogurt
- 1 tsp garlic powder
- 8 slices of whole-grain bread
- 4 slices reduced-fat cheddar cheese

Servings	Prep Time	Cook time
4	10'	6'

COST PER RECIPE	GL
$6	17/ MID

DIRECTIONS

1. In a bowl, combine tuna, Greek yogurt, and garlic powder; mix well.
2. Place 4 slices of bread on a flat surface and divide the tuna mixture evenly over each slice.
3. Top each with 1 slice of cheese and the remaining 4 bread slices.
4. Heat a non-stick skillet over medium heat.
5. Cook the sandwiches 2–3 minutes per side, until the bread is golden and the cheese is melted.
6. Slice and serve warm.

NUTRITION 1 SANDWICH/ SERVING
Calories: 387 kcal | Protein: 36 g | Fat: 9 g | Carbohydrates: 41 g | Fiber: 5 g | Sodium: 412 mg

Creativity TWIST: Add tomato slices under the cheese for extra flavor and moisture without increasing sodium; use multigrain bread for more fiber; or swap cheddar for Swiss for a nuttier flavor without changing carbs.

Hearty Homestyle Vegetable Soup

About this Recipe
Colorful vegetables and tender beans simmer into a simple, satisfying soup that feels wholesome and comforting.

INGREDIENTS

- 15 oz can diced tomatoes, no-salt added
- 15 oz can low-sodium kidney beans, rinsed and drained
- 3 cups of mixed vegetables (fresh or frozen)
- 4 cups low-sodium vegetable broth
- 1 tsp Italian seasoning (no-salt)

DIRECTIONS

1. Add tomatoes, kidney beans, vegetables, and broth to a large soup pot.
2. Stir in Italian seasoning and bring to a boil over medium-high heat.
3. Reduce the heat to low and simmer for 25 minutes, stirring occasionally.
4. Serve warm.

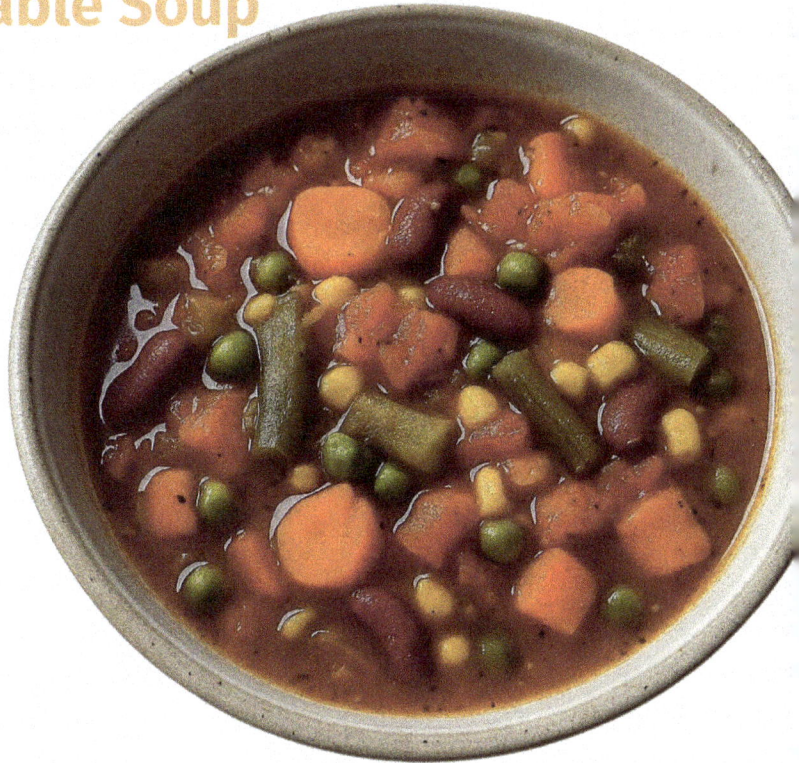

Servings	Prep Time	Cook time
4	10'	25'

GL	COST PER RECIPE
11/ MID	$6

NUTRITION (1 CUP)
Calories: 282 kcal | Protein: 14 g | Fat: 2 g | Carbohydrates: 41 g | Fiber: 13 g | Sodium: 268 mg

Creativity TWIST: Add ½ cup barley or quinoa for extra texture (+6–8 g carbs per serving). For a protein boost, stir in ¼ cup non-fat Greek yogurt before serving instead of sour cream.

Old Fashioned Chicken Noodle Soup

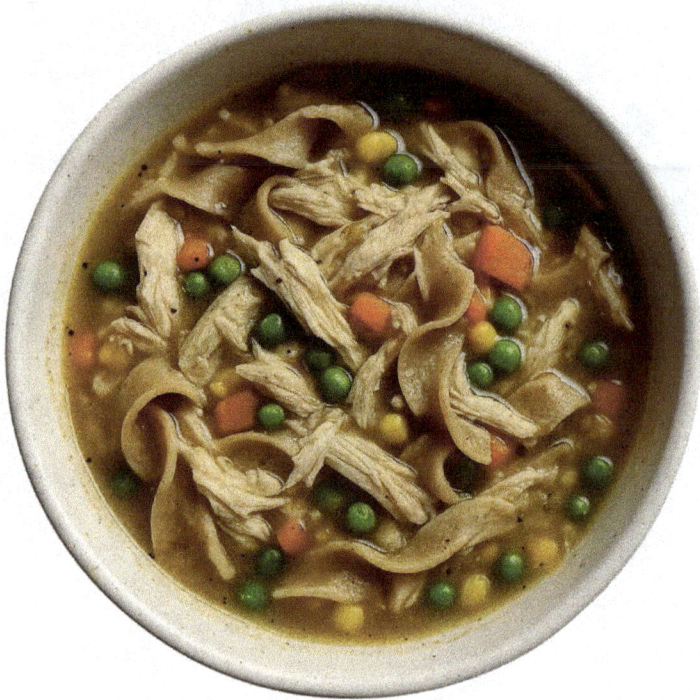

About this Recipe
Warm broth with chicken, noodles, and vegetables creates a simple, cozy soup that comforts with every spoonful.

INGREDIENTS

- 4 cups low-sodium chicken broth
- 2 cups cooked shredded chicken breast
- 2 cups whole-wheat egg noodles (cooked)
- 2 cups frozen mixed vegetables
- 1 tsp Mrs. Dash Table Blend (or homemade salt-free blend)

Servings **4**

Prep Time **10'**

Cook time **20'**

COST PER RECIPE **$6**

GL **13/ MID**

DIRECTIONS

1. Add broth and mixed vegetables to a large soup pot over medium heat.
2. Bring to a light boil, then stir in the shredded chicken and cooked noodles.
3. Season with Mrs. Dash Table Blend and reduce the heat to low.
4. Simmer 10–12 minutes, stirring occasionally.
5. Serve warm (1 cup per serving).

NUTRITION 1 CUP PER SERVING
Calories: 279 kcal | Protein: 31 g | Fat: 5 g | Carbohydrates: 31 g | Fiber: 5 g | Sodium: 240 mg

Creativity TWIST: Add fresh parsley and a squeeze of lemon for brightness without extra sodium; or stir in ¼ cup non-fat Greek yogurt at serving time for extra protein and creaminess.

Crisp Chicken Caesar Salad with Creamy Homemade Caesar Dressing

About this Recipe
Crisp romaine, tender chicken, and creamy Caesar dressing create a fresh, satisfying salad with classic flavor.

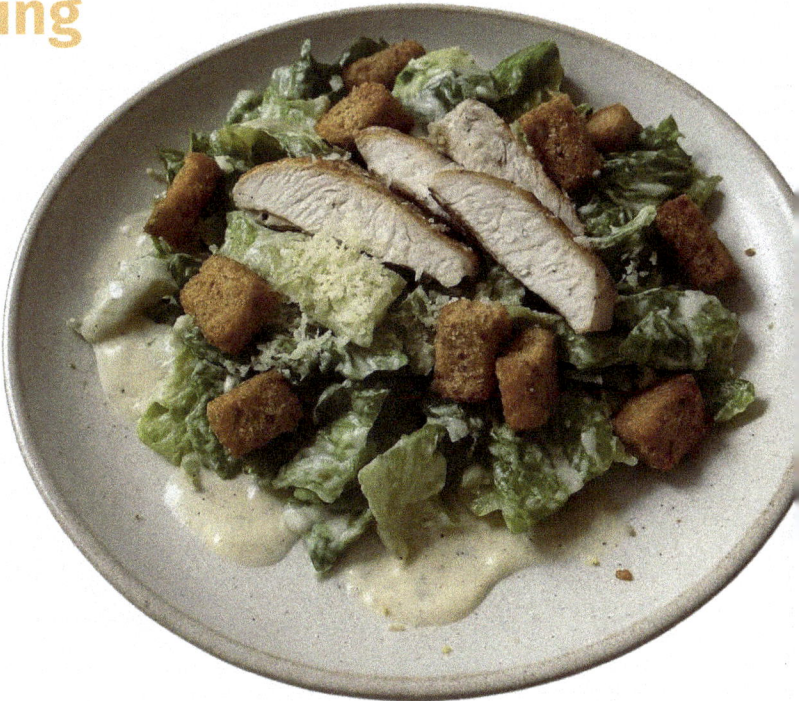

INGREDIENTS

- 4 cups chopped romaine lettuce
- 2 cups cooked sliced chicken breast
- 1 cup whole-wheat croutons
- ½ cup reduced-fat parmesan
- ½ cup non-fat Greek yogurt + ¼ cup grated parmesan + 2 tbsp lemon juice + 1 tbsp Dijon + 1 tbsp Worcestershire (combined = homemade Caesar dressing)

Optional seasonings: minced garlic, black pepper, Italian seasoning

DIRECTIONS

1. Add romaine lettuce to a large bowl and top with sliced chicken, croutons, and parmesan.
2. In a separate bowl, whisk together Greek yogurt, grated parmesan, lemon juice, Dijon mustard, and Worcestershire sauce to make the dressing. Add optional garlic + black pepper to taste.
3. Serve salad with dressing drizzled over the top, or offer dressing on the side so each person can add the amount they prefer.
4. Dressing should be served lightly, not heavily coated.

Servings 4 | Prep Time 15' | Cook time 0'

GL 6/ LOW | COST PER RECIPE $10

NUTRITION (2 CUPS/ SERVING)
Calories: 254 kcal | Protein: 35 g | Fat: 9 g | Carbohydrates: 11 g | Fiber: 2 g | Sodium: 437 mg

Creativity TWIST: Use baked salmon instead of chicken for a seafood Caesar, or add ¼ cup cherry tomatoes for color and extra nutrients without adding sodium.

Hearty Greek Salad with Chickpeas & Feta

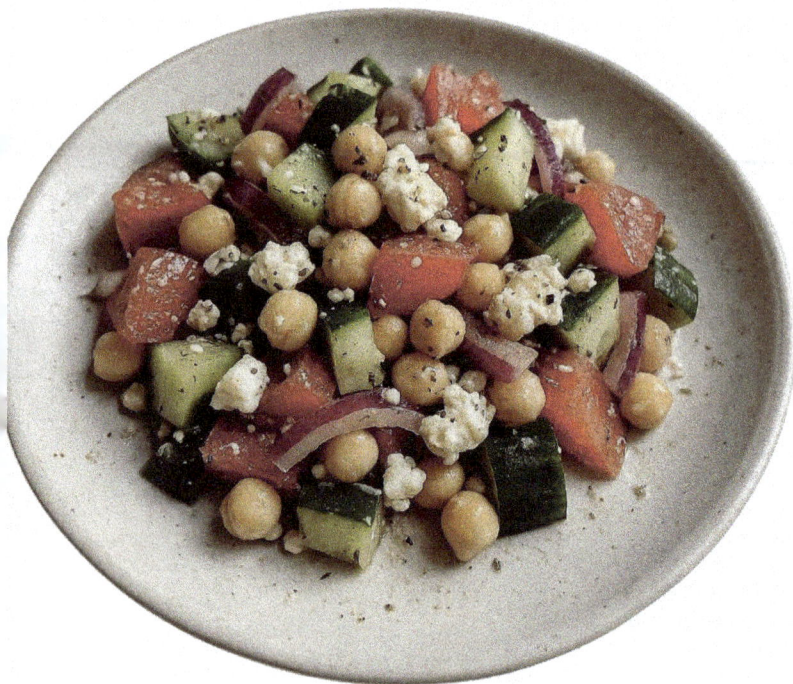

About this Recipe
Cool, crisp veggies with chickpeas and feta create a Mediterranean-style salad that feels hearty, fresh, and filling.

INGREDIENTS

- 4 cups chopped cucumbers + tomatoes + red onion (mixed)
- 1 (15 oz) can chickpeas, rinsed and drained
- ½ cup reduced-fat feta cheese
- 1 tbsp lemon juice
- 1 tsp Italian seasoning (salt-free)
- ½ tsp black pepper

DIRECTIONS

1. Add cucumbers, tomatoes, and red onion to a large bowl.
2. Stir in rinsed chickpeas and feta cheese.
3. Drizzle lemon juice over the top and add Italian seasoning + black pepper.
4. Toss gently to coat and serve chilled.

Servings	Prep Time	Cook time
4	15'	0'

COST PER RECIPE	GL
$8	12/ MID

NUTRITION (2 CUPS PER SERVING)
Calories: 254 kcal | Protein: 35 g | Fat: 9 g | Carbohydrates: 11 g | Fiber: 2 g | Sodium: 437 mg

Creativity TWIST: Add ¼ cup olives only for those not limiting sodium — or add ½ cup spinach for extra volume and fiber without altering the carbs.

Creamy Greek Yogurt with Sugar-Free Pudding

About this Recipe
Creamy, lightly sweet yogurt feels like dessert while delivering a cool, filling, and comforting treat.

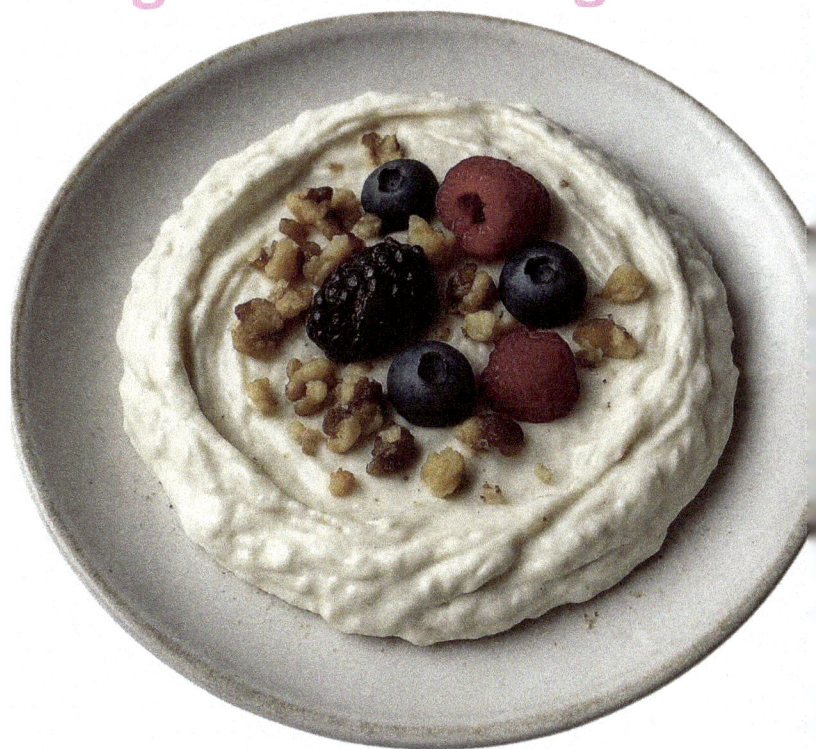

INGREDIENTS

• 3 cups non-fat Greek yogurt
• 1 small box (1 oz) sugar-free instant pudding mix (any flavor)
• ½ cup unsweetened almond milk
• ½ cup berries (fresh or frozen)
• 2 tbsp chopped walnuts
Optional: vanilla extract, cinnamon, sugar-free syrup

DIRECTIONS

1. Add Greek yogurt, instant pudding mix, and almond milk to a mixing bowl.
2. Whisk until smooth and thick (it will thicken more as it rests).
3. Divide evenly into 4 containers (1 cup each).
4. Top with berries and walnuts before serving.
5. Can be refrigerated for up to 4 days.

Servings 4

Prep Time 5'

Cook time 0'

GL 5/ LOW

COST PER RECIPE $9

NUTRITION (1 CUP PER SERVING)
Calories: 239 kcal | Protein: 39 g | Fat: 3.5 g | Carbohydrates: 14 g | Fiber: 2 g | Sodium: 280 mg

Creativity TWIST: Swap berries for sliced peaches or pineapple tidbits (packed in water) for a tropical version — or sprinkle sugar-free chocolate chips for a dessert-style option without adding sodium.

Smooth and Creamy Banana Berry Smoothie

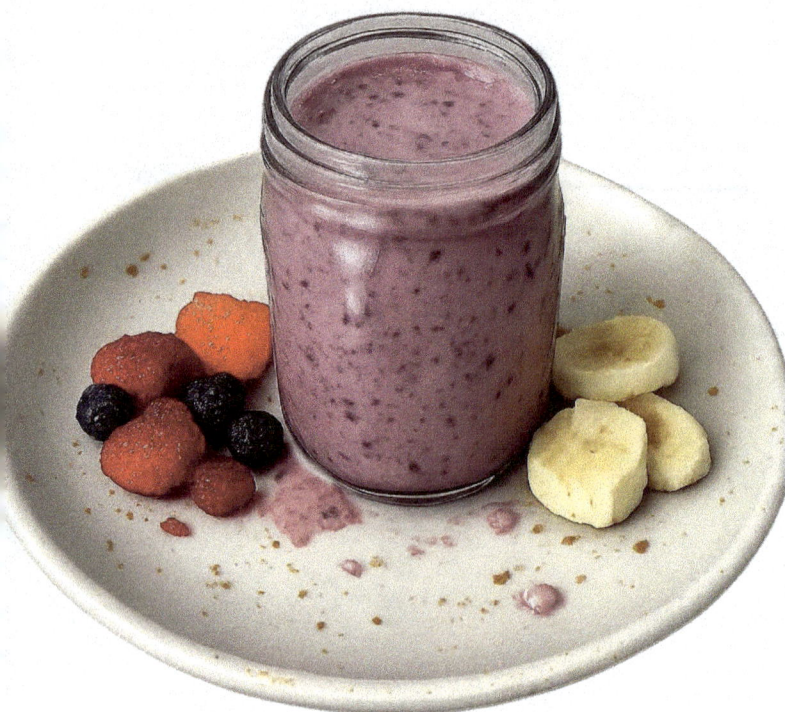

About this Recipe
Cool, fruity, and creamy, this smoothie tastes refreshing and light while feeling smooth and energizing.

INGREDIENTS

- 1 medium banana
- 2 cups frozen mixed berries
- 2 cups unsweetened almond milk
- 1 cup plain non-fat Greek yogurt
- 1 tsp vanilla extract (optional, not counted as ingredient)

DIRECTIONS

1. Add almond milk to blender first.
2. Add banana, berries, Greek yogurt, and vanilla.
3. Blend on high until completely smooth.
4. Add ice if desired and blend until thick and creamy.
5. Pour into 4 glasses and serve immediately.

Servings 4

Prep Time 5'

Cook time 0'

COST PER RECIPE $6

GL 11/ MID

NUTRITION (10 OZ EACH)
Calories: 90 kcal | Protein: 7 g | Fat: 1 g | Carbohydrates: 14 g | Fiber: 2 g | Sodium: 69 mg

Creativity TWIST: For added protein without extra carbs, add 1 scoop vanilla whey isolate or 2 tbsp PB2 powdered peanut butter. For a sweeter taste without added carbs — add ½ packet Splenda or stevia per serving. Freeze leftovers in popsicle molds for a zero-prep frozen dessert.

Warm Sugar-Free Brownie in a Mug

About this Recipe
Warm, fudgy, and rich, this mug brownie delivers cozy chocolate flavor with a satisfying, dessert-like bite.

INGREDIENTS

- 3 tbsp almond flour
- 1 tbsp unsweetened cocoa powder
- 1 scoop chocolate protein powder (sugar-free)
- 1 large egg
- 2 tbsp sugar-free maple syrup

Optional: vanilla extract, cinnamon, sugar-free chocolate chips

DIRECTIONS

1. Add almond flour, cocoa powder, and protein powder to a microwave-safe mug; stir.
2. Add egg and sugar-free maple syrup; mix until smooth with no dry pockets.
3. Microwave 60–75 seconds, depending on microwave strength.
4. Allow to cool 1–2 minutes for the best texture.
5. Serve warm.

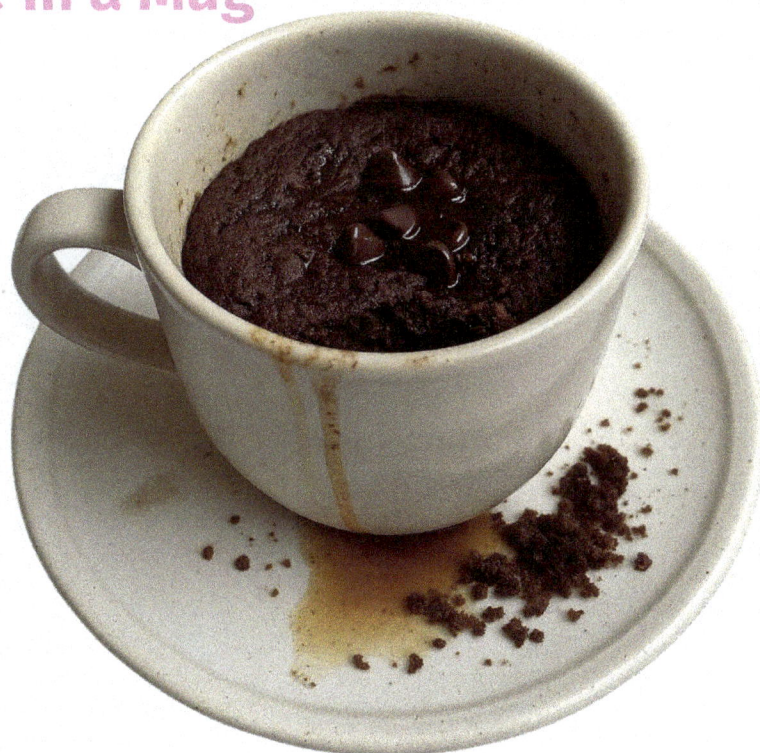

Servings	Prep Time	Cook time
1	3'	60"

GL	COST PER RECIPE
9/LOW	$3

NUTRITION SERVING 1 MUG CAKE
Calories: 234 kcal | Protein: 32 g | Fat: 8 g | Carbohydrates: 14 g | Fiber: 4 g | Sodium: 263 mg

Creativity TWIST: For a molten-center version, microwave for only 50 seconds, add 1 tsp sugar-free chocolate chips in the center, and heat for 15 more seconds.

Creamy Sweet Strawberry Mousse

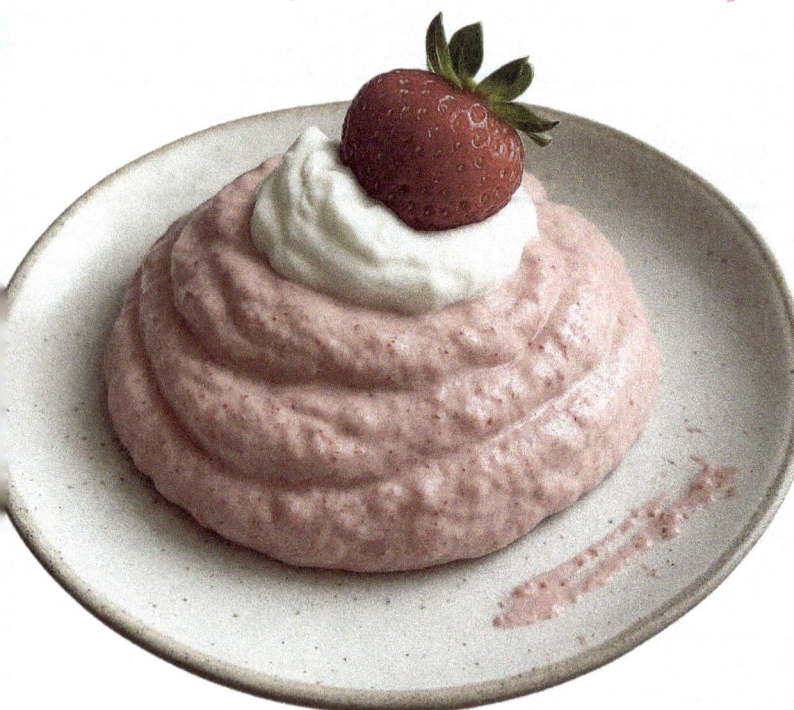

About this Recipe
Light, creamy strawberry mousse tastes sweet and refreshing, feeling indulgent while staying light and satisfying.

INGREDIENTS

- 2 cups frozen strawberries (slightly thawed)
- 2 cups non-fat Greek yogurt
- 2 scoops vanilla protein powder (sugar-free preferred)
- ¼ cup sugar-free maple syrup
- 1 tsp vanilla extract (counts as an ingredient — not a seasoning)

Optional: cinnamon, 4 tbsp light whipped topping for garnish

Servings: 4
Prep Time: 8'
Cook time: 0'
COST PER RECIPE: $8
GL: 6/ LOW

NUTRITION (½ CUP EACH)
Calories: 239 kcal | Protein: 35 g | Fat: 2 g | Carbohydrates: 19 g | Fiber: 3 g | Sodium: 341 mg

Creativity TWIST: Swap strawberries for mango and add coconut flakes for a tropical version, or blend with ½ banana + cocoa powder for a chocolate-covered strawberry flavor without adding sodium.

DIRECTIONS

1. Add strawberries, Greek yogurt, protein powder, vanilla extract, and sugar-free syrup to a blender or food processor.
2. Blend until smooth and fluffy, scraping down the sides as needed.
3. Spoon into 4 small bowls (½ cup each).
4. Chill 30 minutes for the thickest texture (optional).
5. Serve cold.

Chewy Chocolate Banana Oat Cookies

About this Recipe

Soft, chewy cookies with banana sweetness and chocolatey bites taste cozy, comforting, and naturally satisfying.

INGREDIENTS

- 2 cups old-fashioned oats
- 3 ripe bananas, mashed
- ½ cup mini sugar-free chocolate chips

Optional: cinnamon, vanilla extract, 1 tbsp peanut butter powder

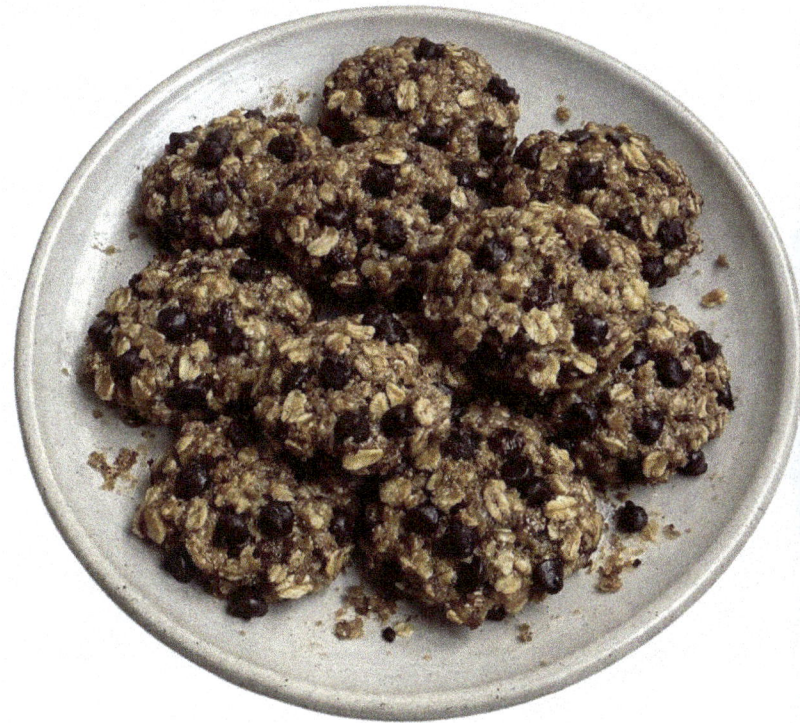

DIRECTIONS

1. Preheat oven to 350°F (177°C) and line a baking sheet with parchment paper.
2. In a bowl, mash bananas until smooth.
3. Stir in oats and chocolate chips until well combined.
4. Scoop dough into 12 cookies (about 2 tbsp each) and place on baking sheet.
5. Bake 12–14 minutes, or until firm and lightly golden.
6. Cool for 5 minutes — serving size = 2 cookies.

Servings
6

Prep Time
8'

Cook time
12'

GL
14/ MID

COST PER RECIPE
$4

NUTRITION (2 COOKIES PER SERVING)
Calories: 173 kcal | Protein: 4 g | Fat: 6 g | Carbohydrates: 32 g | Fiber: 7 g | Sodium: 54 mg

Creativity TWIST: For a molten-center version, microwave for only 50 seconds, add 1 tsp sugar-free chocolate chips in the center, and heat for 15 more seconds.

Spiced Pumpkin Cream Cup

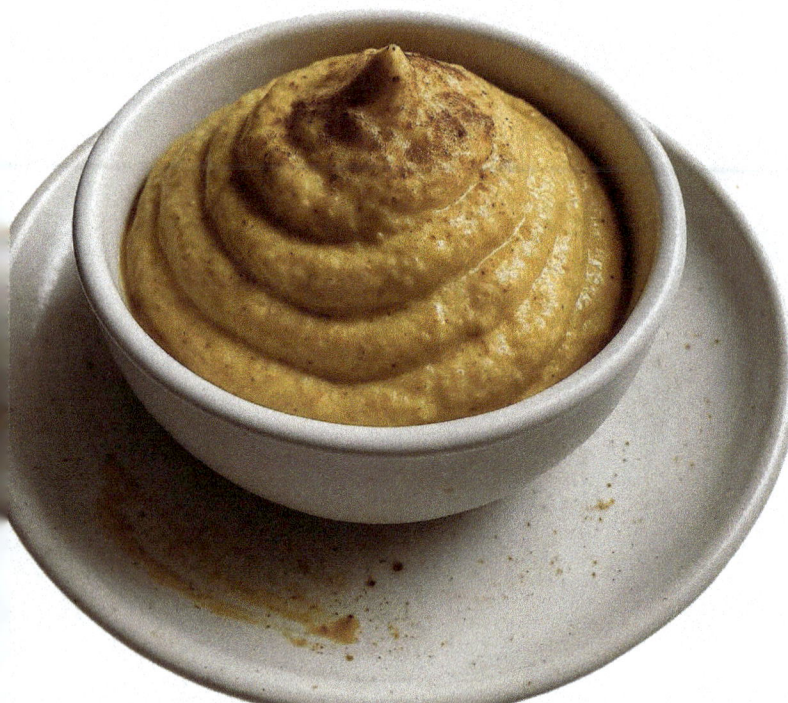

About this Recipe
Cool, spiced pumpkin cream tastes like a fall dessert, feeling smooth, cozy, and lightly indulgent.

INGREDIENTS

- 2 cups frozen banana slices
- 1 cup canned pumpkin puree (plain, not pie mix)
- 1 cup non-fat Greek yogurt
- 2 scoops vanilla protein powder (sugar-free preferred)
- 2 tsp pumpkin pie spice (counts as 1 ingredient — spices do NOT count toward cost)

Optional: splash of almond milk to thin if needed, Splenda if additional sweetness desired

Servings 4
Prep Time 5'
Cook time 0'
COST PER RECIPE $7
GL 8/ LOW

NUTRITION (½ CUP EACH)
Calories: 193 kcal | Protein: 25 g | Fat: 2 g | Carbohydrates: 20 g | Fiber: 4 g | Sodium: 153 mg

Creativity TWIST: Turn it into Pumpkin Cheesecake Dessert by adding 2 tbsp non-fat cream cheese before blending. Or sprinkle 2 tbsp crushed graham cracker crumbs on top for a fall pie flavor while keeping carbs reasonable.

DIRECTIONS

1. Add frozen banana slices, pumpkin puree, Greek yogurt, protein powder, and pumpkin pie spice to a blender or food processor.
2. Blend until smooth and creamy, scraping down the sides as needed.
3. Serve immediately for a soft-serve texture, or freeze for 15–20 minutes for a firmer ice cream texture.
4. Serving size = ½ cup.

Whole-Grain Crackers with Savory Tuna Salad

About this Recipe
Creamy tuna salad with crunchy whole-grain crackers delivers a savory, satisfying snack with great texture.

INGREDIENTS

- 1 (5 oz) can tuna in water, drained
- ¼ cup non-fat Greek yogurt
- 1 tbsp light mayonnaise
- 2 tbsp diced celery
- 24 whole-grain crackers

Optional: black pepper, onion powder, lemon juice, dill

DIRECTIONS

1. In a bowl, combine tuna, Greek yogurt, mayonnaise, and celery.
2. Mix until creamy, season with optional black pepper or dill.
3. Divide the tuna salad into 4 equal portions.
4. Serve each portion with 6 whole-grain crackers.
5. 1 snack = tuna mixture + 6 crackers.

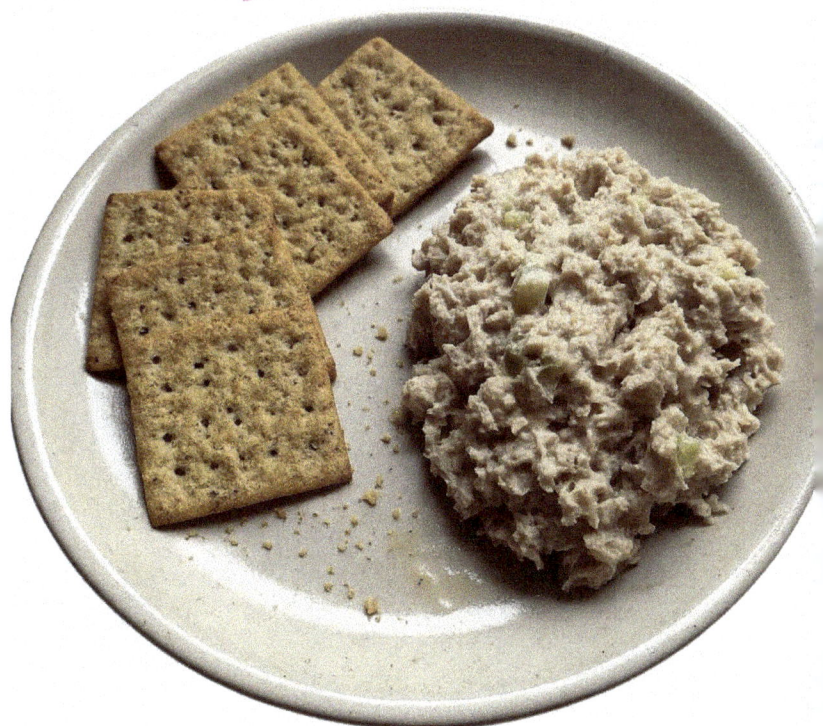

Servings 4 | Prep Time 5' | Cook time 0'

GL 12/ MID | COST PER RECIPE $5

NUTRITION 2 TBSP. TUNA+6 CRACKERS
Calories: 193 kcal | Protein: 9 g | Fat: 3 g | Carbohydrates: 18 g | Fiber: 2 g | Sodium: 416 mg

Creativity TWIST: Swap celery for diced cucumber for extra crunch, or sprinkle in 1 tsp pickle relish for a classic tuna salad flavor without significantly raising sodium.

Homestyle Hummus with Fresh Veggies

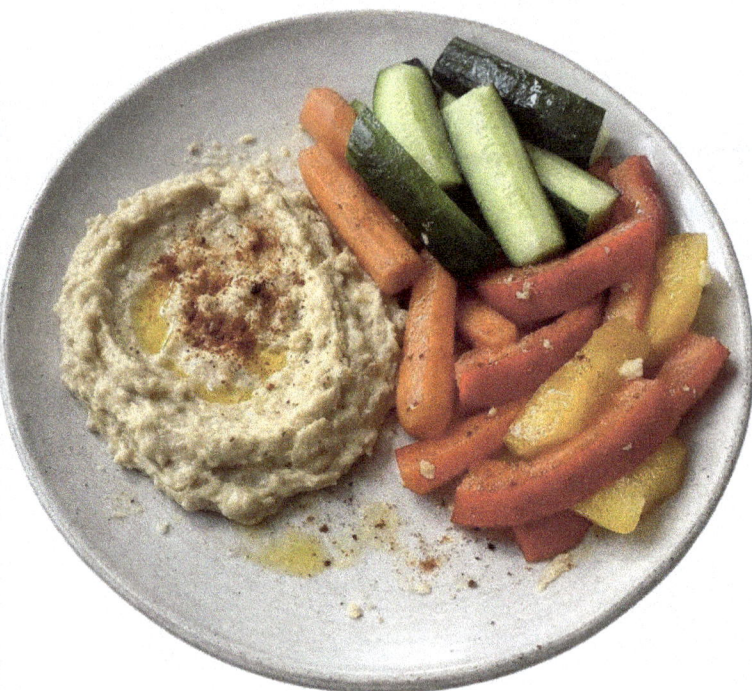

About this Recipe
Creamy, mildly spiced hummus with crisp veggies delivers fresh flavor, satisfying crunch, and a light, filling bite.

Servings
4

Prep Time
8'

Cook time
0'

COST PER RECIPE
$5

GL
8/ LOW

NUTRITION ¼ CUP HUMMUS + 1 CUP VEGGIES
Calories: 198 kcal | **Protein:** 9 g | **Fat:** 5 g | **Carbohydrates:** 27 g | **Fiber:** 6 g | **Sodium:** 166 mg

Creativity TWIST: Replace cumin with everything-but-the-bagel seasoning for a fun variation, or swap Greek yogurt with cottage cheese to increase protein per serving.

INGREDIENTS

- 1 (15 oz) can low-sodium chickpeas, drained & rinsed
- ¼ cup non-fat Greek yogurt
- 1 tbsp olive oil
- 1 tsp cumin (seasoning — does not count toward ingredient limit or cost)
- 4 cups raw mixed vegetables (carrots, cucumbers, bell peppers)

Optional: garlic powder, black pepper, paprika, lemon juice

DIRECTIONS

1. Add chickpeas, Greek yogurt, olive oil, and cumin to a blender or food processor.
2. Blend until smooth; add 1–2 tbsp water only if needed for texture.
3. Portion hummus into 4 containers (¼ cup each).
4. Add 1 cup raw vegetables to each container.
5. 1 snack = ¼ cup hummus + 1 cup mixed vegetables.

Easy Turkey & Cheddar Roll-Ups

About this Recipe
Savory turkey, melty cheddar, and fresh veggies roll into an easy, satisfying snack with great flavor.

INGREDIENTS

8 slices low-sodium deli turkey
• 4 slices reduced-fat cheddar, cut in half
• 1 cup baby spinach leaves
• 4 tbsp light mayonnaise
• 8 grape tomatoes (1 tomato per roll-up)
Optional: black pepper, garlic powder, onion powder, mustard

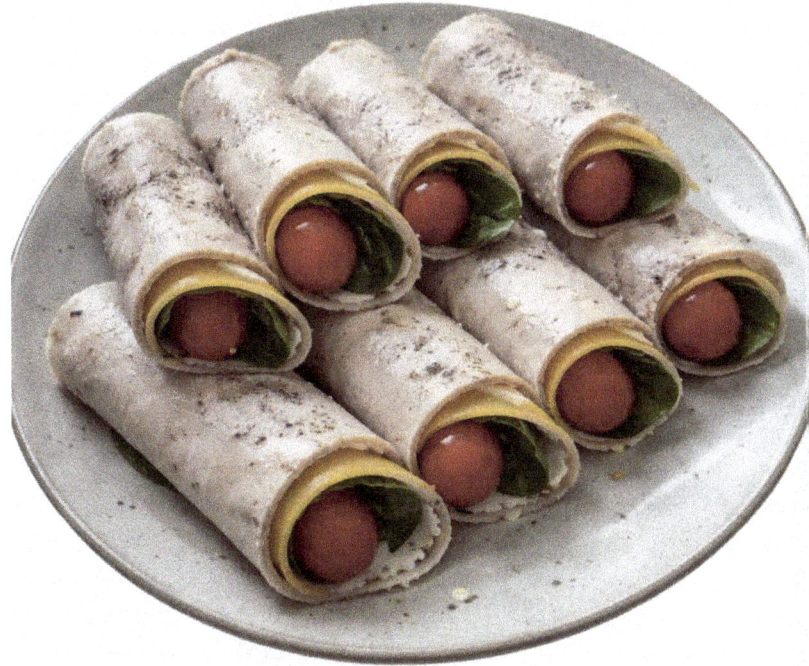

Servings 4 | Prep Time 5' | Cook time 0'

GL 2/ LOW | COST PER RECIPE $8

DIRECTIONS

1. Lay turkey slices flat on a clean surface.
2. Spread ½ tbsp mayonnaise onto each slice.
3. Add 1 half-slice of cheddar + a few spinach leaves + 1 grape tomato to each.
4. Roll up tightly from the short end and place seam-side down.
5. Serve 2 roll-ups per snack serving.

NUTRITION 2 ROLL-UPS
Calories: 166 kcal | Protein: 16 g | Fat: 8 g | Carbohydrates: 7 g | Fiber: 1 g | Sodium: 328 mg

Creativity TWIST: Swap cheddar for Swiss to lower sodium even more, or replace spinach with sliced cucumbers for extra crunch without added carbs

Sweet & Salty Protein Popcorn

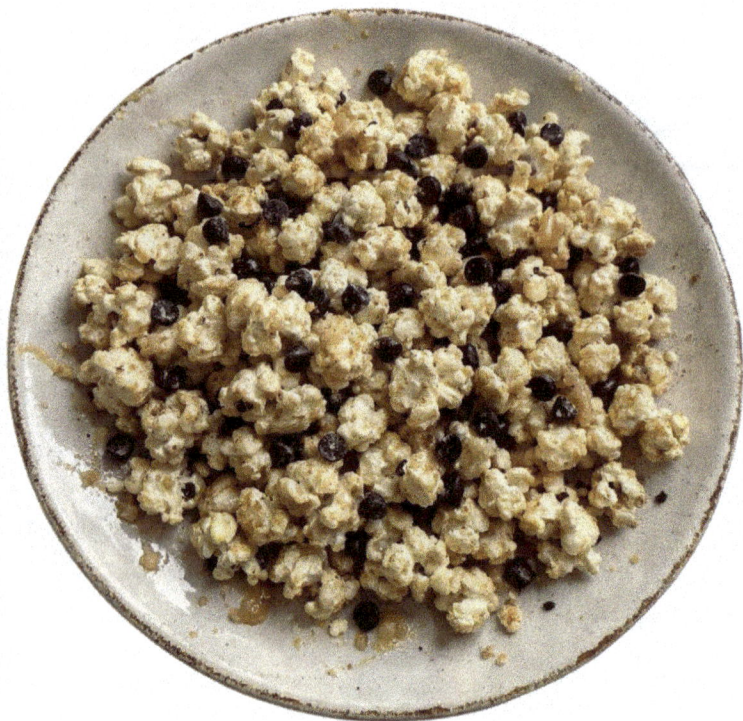

Servings	Prep Time	Cook time
4	5'	60"

COST PER RECIPE	GL
$6	10/ MID

NUTRITION SERVING 2 CUPS
Calories: 171 kcal | Protein: 13 g | Fat: 5 g | Carbohydrates: 23 g | Fiber: 7 g | Sodium: 128 mg

Creativity TWIST: Swap chocolate chips for raisins for a movie-night version (adds 4 g carbs), or add ½ scoop vanilla protein powder to the yogurt mix for an even higher-protein snack.

About this Recipe
Light, crunchy popcorn coated in sweet-salty drizzle delivers a fun, craveable snack that satisfies.

INGREDIENTS

8 cups air-popped popcorn (unsalted)
- ½ cup powdered peanut butter (PB2)
- ½ cup non-fat Greek yogurt
- ¼ cup sugar-free maple syrup
- ¼ cup mini sugar-free chocolate chips

Optional: cinnamon, vanilla extract, a pinch of salt substitute

DIRECTIONS

1. Pop popcorn and allow it to cool slightly.
2. In a bowl, mix powdered peanut butter + Greek yogurt + sugar-free syrup until smooth.
3. Drizzle mixture over popcorn and toss until coated.
4. Fold in sugar-free chocolate chips.
5. Divide into 4 containers — each serving = 2 cups.

Conclusion – A Final Word

You've just reached the end of this Five-Ingredient Diabetes Cookbook, and I hope you're feeling something important right now: confidence.

Confidence that eating well with diabetes does not have to be complicated.

Confidence that balanced, blood-sugar-friendly meals can still be flavorful, satisfying, and realistic for everyday life.

And confidence that with just a handful of thoughtfully chosen ingredients, you can nourish your body without feeling overwhelmed.

Throughout this cookbook, you've learned how simple combinations of lean protein, smart carbohydrates, healthy fats, and fiber can work together to support steady blood sugars without sacrificing taste or enjoyment. These recipes were created to meet you where you are: busy days, limited time, and real-life kitchens. If you found yourself thinking, "I can actually do this," then this book has done its job.

I also hope these recipes have reminded you that diabetes management isn't about perfection. It's about progress, consistency, and confidence in your choices. Whether you're newly diagnosed or have been managing diabetes for years, these meals are meant to be flexible tools you can return to again and again.

Staying Connected

If you'd like more recipes, meal ideas, and diabetes-friendly nutrition tips, I'd love to stay in touch. You can find me online at www.TheDiabetesRDN.com, where I share evidence-based guidance, practical resources, and encouragement to help make diabetes care feel more manageable and less stressful. You'll also find ways to reach out, explore additional cookbooks and tools, and stay connected through newsletters and social media.

One Last Encouragement

Keep experimenting. Keep learning. Keep choosing foods that support your health and your happiness. Small steps, like the ones you've practiced in this cookbook, add up to meaningful, lasting change.

Thank you for welcoming these recipes into your kitchen and for taking another step toward eating well with diabetes.

Warmly,

Elizabeth Berkey, MS, RDN, LD, CDCES, BC-ADM

TheDiabetesRDN

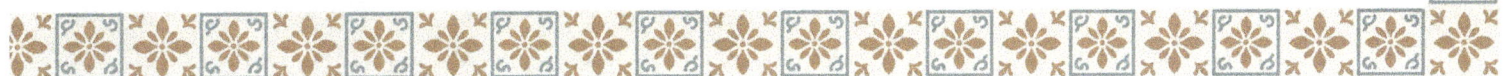

How helpful is this book to you?

I'd love to hear what you think.

I personally read every review, and your feedback means the world to me.It only takes 30 seconds to leave a reivew.

It truly makes a huge difference for a small author like me—and it helps other Diabetes warriors discover this book too.

Here's how you can leave a review for the paperback:

- **Option 1: Go to your Amazon orders, find this book, and click "Write a product review."**

- **Option 2: Scan the QR code to go straight to the review page.**

- **Option 3: Search for the book title on Amazon, scroll down to the "Customer Reviews" section, and click "Write a Review."**

Once you're there, choose a star rating, a quick story about your experience, and submit!

That's it!

Thank you so much // MARIANNE <3

Claim your Bonuses!

◊ Avoid Sugar Spikes - (Carb Swap Cheat Sheet PDF)

◊ Make your own meal plan & adjust recipes (Printable DIY meal plan PDF)

◊ 11 Tips on Staying Active Safely With Diabetes PDF

◊ Get our next book for free as an advanced reader! (via email)

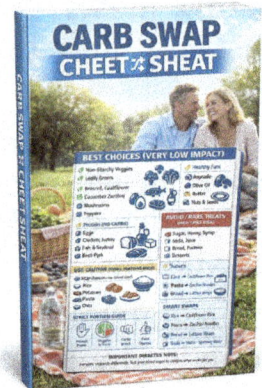

Grab your Copy of "the Diabetes Reset" by scanning the QR below!

Your simple guide to understand the root causes of Diabetes

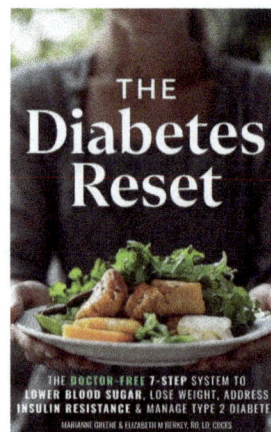

Conclusion – A Final Word

You've just reached the end of this Five-Ingredient Diabetes Cookbook, and I hope you're feeling something important right now: confidence.

Confidence that eating well with diabetes does not have to be complicated.

Confidence that balanced, blood-sugar-friendly meals can still be flavorful, satisfying, and realistic for everyday life.

And confidence that with just a handful of thoughtfully chosen ingredients, you can nourish your body without feeling overwhelmed.

Throughout this cookbook, you've learned how simple combinations of lean protein, smart carbohydrates, healthy fats, and fiber can work together to support steady blood sugars without sacrificing taste or enjoyment. These recipes were created to meet you where you are: busy days, limited time, and real-life kitchens. If you found yourself thinking, "I can actually do this," then this book has done its job.

I also hope these recipes have reminded you that diabetes management isn't about perfection. It's about progress, consistency, and confidence in your choices. Whether you're newly diagnosed or have been managing diabetes for years, these meals are meant to be flexible tools you can return to again and again.

Staying Connected

If you'd like more recipes, meal ideas, and diabetes-friendly nutrition tips, I'd love to stay in touch. You can find me online at www.TheDiabetesRDN.com, where I share evidence-based guidance, practical resources, and encouragement to help make diabetes care feel more manageable and less stressful. You'll also find ways to reach out, explore additional cookbooks and tools, and stay connected through newsletters and social media.

One Last Encouragement

Keep experimenting. Keep learning. Keep choosing foods that support your health and your happiness. Small steps, like the ones you've practiced in this cookbook, add up to meaningful, lasting change.

Thank you for welcoming these recipes into your kitchen and for taking another step toward eating well with diabetes.

Warmly,

Elizabeth Berkey, MS, RDN, LD, CDCES, BC-ADM

TheDiabetesRDN

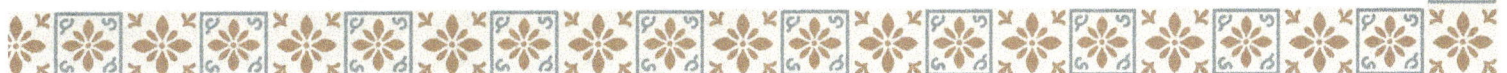

How helpful is this book to you?

I'd love to hear what you think.

I personally read every review, and your feedback means the world to me.It only takes 30 seconds to leave a reivew.

It truly makes a huge difference for a small author like me—and it helps other Diabetes warriors discover this book too.

Here's how you can leave a review for the paperback:

- **Option 1: Go to your Amazon orders, find this book, and click "Write a product review."**

- **Option 2: Scan the QR code to go straight to the review page.**

- **Option 3: Search for the book title on Amazon, scroll down to the "Customer Reviews" section, and click "Write a Review."**

Once you're there, choose a star rating, a quick story about your experience, and submit!

That's it!

Thank you so much // MARIANNE <3

Claim your Bonuses!

◊ Avoid Sugar Spikes - (Carb Swap Cheat Sheet PDF)

◊ Make your own meal plan & adjust recipes (Printable DIY meal plan PDF)

◊ 11 Tips on Staying Active Safely With Diabetes PDF

◊ Get our next book for free as an advanced reader! (via email)

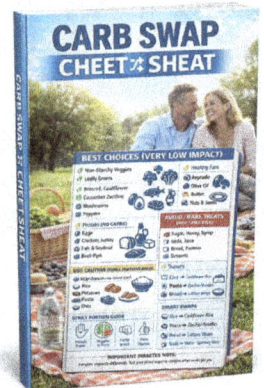

Grab your Copy of "the Diabetes Reset" by scanning the QR below!

Your simple guide to understand the root causes of Diabetes

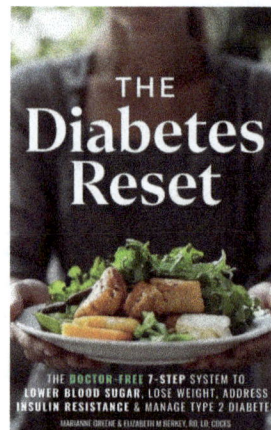

Resources

Start here (beginner-friendly, trusted)

◊ ADA – Food & Nutrition (meal planning basics): https://diabetes.org/food-nutrition (American Diabetes Association)

◊ CDC – Type 2 Diabetes (overview, symptoms, prevention): https://www.cdc.gov/diabetes/about/about-type-2-diabetes.html (CDC)

◊ NIDDK – Healthy Living with Diabetes (practical day-to-day guide): https://www.niddk.nih.gov/health-information/diabetes/overview/healthy-living-with-diabetes (NIDDK)

◊ MedlinePlus – Type 2 Diabetes (NIH-reviewed basics + links): https://medlineplus.gov/diabetestype2.html (MedlinePlus)

Meal planning + low-effort cooking (fits your 5-ingredient/30-min niche)

◊ ADA – "Plan Your Plate" (portion method PDF): https://professional.diabetes.org/sites/dpro/files/2025-05/PE25-Plan-Your-Plate-FINAL-5-22-25.pdf (professional.diabetes.org)

◊ CDC – Diabetes Meal Planning (tools + booklet links): https://www.cdc.gov/diabetes/healthy-eating/diabetes-meal-planning.html (CDC)

◊ USDA SNAP-Ed Recipes (healthy + thrifty recipes): https://snaped.fns.usda.gov/resources/recipes-and-menus/snap-ed-recipes (snaped.fns.usda.gov)

◊ ADA Diabetes Food Hub – Meal Planner ("Plan My Meals"): https://diabetesfoodhub.org/plan-my-meals (diabetesfoodhub.org)

Carbs, labels, and smart swaps (core beginner skills)

◊ ADA – Reading Food Labels (diabetes-focused): https://diabetes.org/food-nutrition/reading-food-labels/making-sense-food-labels (American Diabetes Association)

◊ FDA – How to Use the Nutrition Facts Label: https://www.fda.gov/food/nutrition-facts-label/how-understand-and-use-nutrition-facts-label (U.S. Food and Drug Administration)

◊ ADA – Understanding Carbs: https://diabetes.org/food-nutrition/understanding-carbs (American Diabetes Association)

◊ Diabetes Canada – Glycemic Index Food Guide: https://www.diabetes.ca/managing-my-diabetes/tools---resources/glycemic-index-%28gi%29-food-guide (diabetes.ca)

Evidence-based research (for "go deeper" readers + author research)

◊ ADA – Standards of Care (clinical guidelines hub): https://

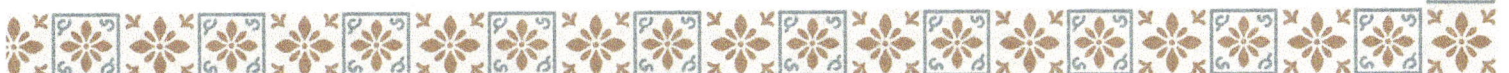

professional.diabetes.org/standards-of-care (professional.diabetes.org)

◊ PubMed (search medical research papers): https://pubmed.ncbi.nlm.nih.gov/ (PubMed)

◊ Cochrane Library (high-quality evidence reviews): https://www.cochranelibrary.com/ (cochranelibrary.com)

◊ ClinicalTrials.gov (ongoing studies + results): https://clinicaltrials.gov/ (ClinicalTrials.gov)

Support + programs (education that improves outcomes)

◊ CDC – Find a DSMES Program (diabetes education & support): https://www.cdc.gov/diabetes/education-support-programs/find-a-dsmes-program.html (CDC)

◊ ADCES – Find an Accredited Diabetes Education Program: https://www.adces.org/program-finder (ADCES)

◊ CBDCE – Locate a CDCES (find a diabetes education specialist): https://www.cbdce.org/locate (CBDCE)

◊ CDC – Find a National DPP Lifestyle Change Program (prediabetes/early prevention): https://www.cdc.gov/diabetes-prevention/lifestyle-change-program/find-a-program.html (CDC)

Tools & apps (tracking helps beginners stay consistent)

◊ mySugr (log glucose/meals/meds): https://www.mysugr.com/ (mySugr)

References from the Introduction part

◊ American Diabetes Association. (2019). Nutrition Therapy for Adults With Diabetes or Prediabetes: A Consensus Report. Diabetes Care, 42(5), 731–754.

◊ American Diabetes Association. (2024). Checking your blood sugar. https://diabetes.org/health-wellness/checking-your-blood-sugar

◊ Brock, K. (2020). Glycemic Index (GI) or Glycemic Load (GL) and Dietary Interventions: A Review. Nutrition, 145, 111577.

◊ Reynolds, A. (2024). Dietary Advice for Individuals with Diabetes. Endotext, NCBI Bookshelf.

◊ American Heart Association. (2023). Added Sugars and Cardiometabolic Risk.

◊ Brock, K. (2020). Glycemic Index (GI) or Glycemic Load (GL) and Dietary Interventions: A Review. Nutrition, 145, 111577

◊ American Diabetes Association. (n.d.). Reading food labels: Making sense of food labels.

◊ https://diabetes.org/food-nutrition/reading-food-labels/making-sense-food-labels